FEET FIRST

Barefoot Performance and Hoof
Rehabilitation

FEET FIRST

Barefoot Performance and Hoof Rehabilitation

NIC BARKER and
SARAH BRAITHWAITE

J. A. ALLEN · LONDON

© Nic Barker and Sarah Braithwaite, 2009
First published in Great Britain 2009

ISBN 978 0 85131 960 5

J.A. Allen
Clerkenwell House
Clerkenwell Green
London ECIR OHT

www.halebooks.com

J. A. Allen is an imprint of Robert Hale Limited

A catalogue record for this book is available from the British Library

Extracts from *The Nature of Horses* by Stephen Budiansky are reproduced by permission of
Orion Publishing Group Ltd., extracts from *No Foot, No Horse* by M. Deacon and G. Williams
are reproduced by permission of Kenilworth Press. The quotation from *Bad Medicine*
by David Wootton is reproduced by permission of Oxford University Press.

Edited by Lesley Gowers and Martin Diggle
Designed and typeset by Paul Saunders

Photographs by the authors, except for those on page 48 (Mathew Jackson), page 59
(Mark Johnson), page 76 (Action Shots Photography www.actionshots.me.uk),
page 77 upper (Kirt Lander), lower and jacket photo of Sarah and Jesta (West End
Photography), pages 78 and 155 (Fotograffs), page 107 (Corrie Curtis/Nathan Shallcross),
page 153 (NaturalScape Countryside and Event Photography) and page 158
(www.joannaprestwich.co.uk).

Illustrations by Carole Viner

Printed in China and arranged by New Era Printing Co. Ltd

Contents

Foreword

When people from different countries, backgrounds and beliefs begin to walk a broadly similar path; when certified, skilled professionals put part of their tool kit to one side in favour of what nature has already provided, is it not the obvious and intelligent response to ask why?

I began working actively with horse's feet when I was 14 and at the time of writing this I am 46 and a registered UK farrier. In my earlier years could I have imagined that herbs and minerals might in some cases replace the need for shoes and nails? Would I ever have guessed that a good practice of regular and sufficient exercise might in some cases replace the need for me to worry myself over hoof balance, instead allowing muscles to develop and carry the skeleton as nature had intended?

My focused involvement with the 'barefoot' movement came through an introduction to Nic Barker and Sarah Braithwaite, both co-founder members of the UKNHCP and co-authors of this book. I was already involved in actively supporting horses and owners who wanted to remain shoeless and was giving a talk to a group of horse owners on the subject. Nic and Sarah came along to that talk, to find out where I was coming from and in return I asked them to look at a horse for me which I couldn't fix.

This was my first introduction to holistic hoofcare, and how naïve it seems to me now that, without placing whole body health at the very top of the agenda, the likelihood of success was much more limited. As a farrier who still shoes horses, it is now essential that I use the knowledge that I have gained from the barefoot movement. I had never appreciated just how sick many of the horses that I was dealing with were and are. Whether shod or shoeless, health is everything. This is not meant to sound as if I am trying to replace veterinary advice, far from it. The difference is that veterinary training is quite rightly science-based and new scientific ideas take time to be properly reviewed.

The barefoot world is incredibly dynamic; if a good working solution is discovered, it is normally circulated very quickly across a vast number of horses, giving rise to a massively broad field trial. Although anecdotal, the evidence (whether good or bad) rapidly becomes self-evident.

So, what would I wish for the future? I would wish that, for the sake of equine welfare, the barefoot movement continues to grow and takes its rightful place as one of the prime educators for domestic horse-keeping throughout the world. I would wish especially that my profession of farriery will move forward to embrace the information, which is so generously available and so beneficial to the horse which we serve, as part of its training.

Mark Johnson DipWCF
March 2009

Acknowledgements

This book is the result of the years we have spent observing and analysing horses and their hooves. Many people have helped us along the way – too many to mention here – but the following are a few who have been invaluable, and whom we'd like to thank publicly.

Pete Ramey, who provided our initial inspiration and encouragement and spurred us on to what has become a passion.

Dr Robert Bowker VMD PhD, whose constant work in comparing 'good' and 'bad' hooves has provided ground-breaking research, and answers to many of our questions.

Our wonderful farriers, Matthew Jackson DipWCF, Mark Johnson DipWCF and Paul Jackson RSS who helped us found the UK Natural Hoof Care Practitioners (UKNHCP), for their support and willingness to stick their heads above the parapet with us on numerous occasions. They have equalled our passion for hooves and added to our knowledge through their years of experience with farriery.

Our partners, Andy Willis and Lee Proctor, for the patience they have shown while we have embarked upon an (at times obsessive) quest for answers about hooves, and then spent long hours in discussion. Without their understanding and, at times, unbelievable tolerance, we would never have been able to gather the knowledge to write this book.

Finally, and most importantly, the horses, the ultimate experts on the hoof: not just our own horses but the hundreds of clients' horses who have each added something to our understanding of how their hooves mirror their health.

Authors' note

This book is written in the full knowledge that the only rule that applies to horses is *'sometimes, but not always'*, and for every generalisation in this book there will be at least one horse for whom the opposite is true.

Introduction

Welcome

We have ridden and competed our own horses barefoot for over ten years. Between us we have taken many hundreds of our clients' horses out of shoes and helped their owners to work them barefoot. These horses work in almost every discipline and their owners tried natural hoof care for different reasons.

Some horses had specific problems or lameness, and barefoot was the last resort for them and their owners; some were perfectly sound and their owners were attracted to the philosophy of natural hoof care and wanted their horses to have the healthiest possible feet.

We do not view barefoot as a holy grail. Although we are passionate about helping horses to grow the best functioning hooves, we appreciate that shoes are frequently the most practical option for many owners.

Keeping a horse barefoot is simply a different way of managing your horse's hoof care and it is up to you, the owner, to make an informed choice by being aware of the possibilities and implications of both shoeing and natural hoof care. This book may help you decide whether natural hoof care is the right choice for you and your horse.

If you are new to natural hoof care, then parts of this book may appear surprising, or even controversial. We did not set out to be controversial, but documenting the capabilities of bare hooves means that we are likely to astonish some people.

Indeed, over the years, the incredible ability of the bare equine hoof has astonished us too. Both our own horses and those of our clients continually show us that man has often misunderstood how hooves function and how strong they can become under the right circumstances.

To date, relatively little has been written about barefoot horses in the

UK, especially barefoot performance horses. We hope this book will start to fill that gap, and perhaps lead to more research in the future.

> We use the terms 'natural hoof care', 'barefoot' and 'unshod' throughout this book, and it is perhaps worth explaining what we mean. We are using 'barefoot' and 'natural hoof care' to apply to domestic horses who are working without shoes, whether that is as a Riding Club horse, hack, or high-level competition horse. We use 'unshod' to describe horses who do not have shoes, but who are not in work, such as retired horses, companions, broodmares and young stock. (Further terms are explained in the Glossary.)

We have studied the horse's hoof over many years, and have read farriery and veterinary textbooks and talked to many experts on the hoof, both practitioners and academics; at the end of the day, we always come back to our own and our clients' horses, and they have taught us the most of all. This book therefore is not an academic study, but it is totally evidence-based: everything we have written is the result of years of our own experience of barefoot horses; everything has been tried, tested and proven on horses working and competing without shoes in the UK.*

Where we came from

For quite some time after news of barefoot horses had started to make headlines in the USA, there was a belief that horses could never work without shoes in the UK because our climate is so wet. Actually, there is a huge amount of truth in this myth, but it is not necessarily for the reasons you might think.

Although we initially focused on trimming horses, what we quickly learnt – albeit through trial and error – is that the most important factors that determine hoof health are diet, environment and exercise.

Once our horses were out of shoes, we gained incredible feedback from monitoring how the performance of our horses' hooves changed over time. It became obvious that these changes could be linked to changes in diet, environment and exercise.

We now know that getting these three elements right is the foundation

---

* We, together with other UK Natural Hoof Care Practitioners, vets and farriers, are committed to carrying out more research into natural hoof care, and hoof function generally. Latest research is published via www.uknhcp.org

upon which healthy hooves are built. If any of these elements are out of balance, hooves can become unhealthy and unable to perform.

We've seen over the years that even horses with poor hooves can improve their hoof function and hoof quality given the right diet, environment and exercise. For many horses, getting these elements right will make the difference between lameness and soundness. In fact, it is usually the horses with the worst feet who improve the most once they are barefoot.

Until recently, few people realised how dynamic a horse's hoof really is, how relatively quickly it can be transformed, and what incredible levels of performance a truly healthy hoof is capable of.

This book will show you what constitutes a healthy hoof – what it looks like, how it performs, how it develops, and perhaps most importantly, how you can help your own horse's hooves become healthier.

1

What is a healthy hoof?

A working definition

We have a working definition of a healthy hoof that we use every day to assess our own horses' hooves and our clients' horses' hooves.

Our experience is that a horse with healthy hooves is more than capable of trotting, cantering or galloping over stones, flint or gravel unshod, and of covering this type of ground day in, day out. We therefore use this level of performance as our benchmark – we define a horse with healthy hooves as one who is sound, *without shoes*, over challenging surfaces, at any speed.

The reason we assess hooves using this benchmark so regularly is because the health of hooves can change very quickly.

Of course, very many horses in the UK have hooves that are not as capable as this. For our purposes, we would define these horses as having unhealthy hooves, but the good news is that hooves are dynamic, and even horses with bad hooves can improve them.

Take a look, for instance, at the horse's hoof in the first photo opposite. This shows the state of his hooves only a few days after he came out of shoes. Dexter is an eventer, but he had been lame for some months before this photo was taken and he had been diagnosed with deep digital flexor tendonitis. Remedial shoeing had been unable to improve him, and over time he had become steadily more lame. At the time of this photo, he was noticeably lame when trotted on an even, hard surface in a straight line.

He is a Thoroughbred, and had been described as having 'typical Thoroughbred feet' – in other words, flat feet, with thin, brittle hoof wall and sole, under-run heels and long toes.

The second photo shows his hoof less than four months afterwards, and at this stage he was back in full work. He was sound to trot on the

- Hoof health is a good indicator of overall health of the horse.

- A healthy hoof will engage the back of the foot on landing, with the frog, digital cushion and lateral cartilages able to absorb shock to protect tendons and ligaments.

- The quality of the hoof wall and the sole provide clues to metabolic problems or dietary deficiencies.

- The condition of the frog, heels and digital cushion will highlight biomechanical issues.

- Hooves are dynamic – they can and do change radically as a result of mechanical forces, muscle wastage and dietary deficiencies.

same surface in a straight line, and had started competing again. Although his hoof is far from perfect in the second photo, many of the earlier problems have improved dramatically. His toe is shorter, and his heels less under-run.

In fact his whole hoof is further underneath him, and the structures of his hoof are able to support him better. His frog and heels are stronger, and have de-contracted, and his sole is no longer flat, but has the beginnings of good concavity.

This horse was sound to work on most surfaces, including roads, but he still tended to pick his way over the roughest, stoniest ground. He had shown an incredible improvement from a seriously lame horse, unable to

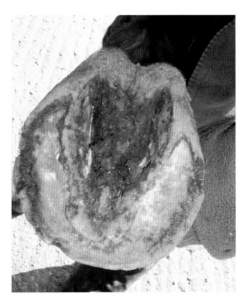 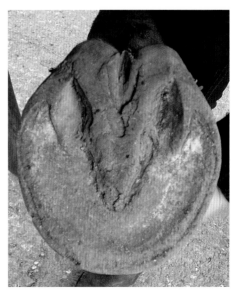

RIGHT Dexter's sole in February.

FAR RIGHT Dexter; the same foot 4 months later.

work, to a horse who could resume a competitive career. Using our bench-mark, though, he did not have the perfect 'healthy hoof' at this stage because he could not stride out confidently over challenging surfaces.

In this relatively short time, his hooves had grown much stronger. Just as it took him many months to become lame, so it will take many months of correct work and stimulus before his hooves become as strong as they could be and reach perfect health.

His hooves demonstrate the amazing ability of the horse's body to grow a better hoof, but they also show that when a hoof (like any other part of the body) has been seriously compromised over many years, it may take equally long to fully recover; in cases of the most serious damage, of course, full recovery may not even be possible.

Belief and proof

We had a very interesting experience hunting on Exmoor one day. There was a group of visiting hunting folk, who had not realised that the two horses we were riding had no shoes.

It wasn't until the end of the day that they noticed that the horses were barefoot. Their belief system was turned upside down by what they were seeing.

They believed that some native ponies could cope without shoes; they believed that horses who did no roadwork could cope without shoes. What they couldn't understand was what they were seeing: they were literally unable to believe their eyes.

They tried to rationalise what they were seeing by asking if our horses were native-bred. The only problem is that our horses didn't look remotely native. One was a Warmblood, the other a lightweight Irish sports horse. They then asked if we were able to cope because we did no roadwork. That idea was confounded as our horses trotted down the road next to them, after more than seven hours out hunting.

Time and time again, we meet people who have been conditioned to believe that horses cannot work without shoes, and who carry on believing that, despite the evidence of their own eyes.

Even we sometimes find it hard to believe just what a healthy hoof can achieve, despite the fact that our horses now prove it to us every day.

2

Why shoes?

What horse owners assumed

Like the vast majority of British horse owners, we had always assumed that horses needed shoes. During more than thirty years of owning horses, we had not questioned this assumption, nor had we ever come across a hard-working barefoot horse.

In fact it had never occurred to either one of us that it might be possible to have a horse who was able to hunt, event, compete in endurance or work on the roads without metal shoes.

The received wisdom throughout our experience of horse-keeping created the belief that horses needed shoes for protection and support in order to do any sort of serious work. The message that you could not keep working horses' feet healthy without the use of horseshoes was one we read and had been taught about time and time again from childhood onwards.

Of course, horses in the wild did not have shoes on but, like everyone else, we believed that our modern roads, combined with the weight of a rider or pulling a vehicle, put such demands on the physiology of the horse that it was impossible for them to function without shoes.

The idea that you had no choice but to shoe was ingrained into our subconscious to such an extent that questioning the practice seemed like complete nonsense. What kind of owners would we be if we allowed stones to become embedded in an unprotected white line, creating the possibility for abscessing or even pedal bone infection? If we took our horses on roads to a greater (or even a lesser) extent, might we not wear the hooves away to stumps, or cause mechanical laminitis?

What the professionals believed

Like most owners, our views had been influenced by what was considered to be the 'received wisdom' of the experts. The belief that horses need shoes to work has perpetuated, without being questioned by any but a tiny minority of horse owners, even up to the present day. It's a belief that had a limpet-like hold on our imaginations, and still retains a limpet-like hold on the imagination of most equine professionals in the UK today.

We had read many standard equine textbooks stating that horses must be shod if they were to be worked on the road. It is interesting that this belief persists even today, when there is ample evidence that horses with healthy feet cope admirably with extensive roadwork, and that, in fact, their feet are even healthier if roadwork is a regular part of their exercise programme.

Nevertheless, old habits and prejudices die hard, and it is still seen as safer to advise that horses be shod.

One point that we had not fully appreciated until a few years ago was that many farriers had their own reservations about shoeing horses, and in many cases viewed shoeing as an invasive act.

Some of the best farriers were, in fact, reluctant to shoe, and even went so far as to state that shoeing over the long term damaged hooves. They were between a rock and a hard place, however, as they could see that shoeing seemed to be a prerequisite if horses were to be able to work.

A guarded, or downright negative view of shoeing was clearly set out in some farriery textbooks. In the early years of the last century, two authorities had expressed the view that shoeing was no better than a necessary evil:

> ...fully 90 per cent of the diseases to which horseflesh is heir can be traced to the driving of nails into the hoof.
>
> *Evolution of the Horse Shoe*, H. D. Shaiffer, 1912

> ...with artificial roads...we are compelled to protect [the hoof] by the use of a shoe, not forgetting that no man improves a foot by shoeing – we may and often do mar it.
>
> *The Care of the Horse*, Professor W. Jones Anstey, FWCF, FZS, 1929

More recently, another book gives more detailed expression to similar reservations:

> Shoeing alters the natural function of the hoof wall...Metal shoes increase the concussive forces transmitted from the hoof to the bones inside the hoof. They are also known to decrease the hoof's natural shock-absorption. This leads to a double-whammy effect – the shoes increase the concussion and at the same time decrease the foot's ability to absorb that concussion.
>
> *No Foot, No Horse*, Gail Williams and Martin Deacon, 2002

So it seems there was a consistent objective amongst leading farriers: how to fit a shoe with the least interference to the horse's natural gait and biomechanics and the least damage to the hoof itself – and this objective had fuelled many of the recent developments in shoeing, such as Natural Balance shoes.

Despite these concerns and reservations, over the years, the consistent message for owners has been that only an uncaring owner would try to make a horse go without shoes, and that such an owner would be likely to cause their horse pain and possibly serious physical damage, which at best might take a long time to heal or at worst could be permanent.

Add to this the belief (still current) that shoes somehow provide the horse with 'support', and that, without a rim of steel around the edge of the hoof, the bony column of the leg will be put under intolerable strain, such that the horse might even break down.

In the case of a horse with less than perfect conformation or movement, the experts say, the hooves on the end of those less than perfect limbs need even more support and protection from the damage of uneven wear.

It is certainly true that many horses in the UK are uncomfortable if they lose a shoe, but miraculously sound once the shoe is replaced, and this is a powerful piece of evidence in favour of the belief that horses need shoes.

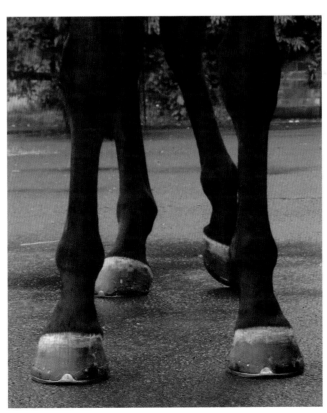

A traditionally shod working horse.

There has always been a minority of horses (actually, more commonly, ponies) who have been able to walk soundly without the protection of shoes, but their hoof walls appeared to chip, flare and crack under their weight once they were on harder ground.

The general consensus of opinion has been that man has bred the hooves out of horses, creating weak, pale inferior specimens in contrast to the hooves of Xenophon's army of war horses. In any case, surely no hoof would be able to withstand the demands of domestication without being shod.

So, fear of the unknown, and a reluctance to challenge convention caused us to be unable to question the practice of shoeing horses, believing that it must be right because it had been carried out for hundreds of years.

By 2008, we had been on our own voyages of discovery for several years and we, along with many other people, had publicised an ever-increasing body of evidence that horses could work hard and compete without shoes. Nevertheless, the UK government's draft equine welfare code was still upholding the tradition:

> Horses ridden or driven on roads or hard, rough surfaces should be regularly shod...
>
> *Draft Code of Practice for the Welfare of Equines*, Welsh/Scottish Assembly, 2007

What the horses told us

Against this background, we inevitably had our own horses shod, and of course we each had horses who were lame and sore as soon as they lost a shoe – a powerful and sensible persuasion for the use of a horseshoe.

Twenty, or even ten, years ago there were a few unshod ponies being worked but, as a rule, if you did not shoe your horse, it was because you were either unable or unwilling to pay a farrier or find a farrier, or because you had a horse who would not tolerate being shod. The overriding assumption was that if you did not shoe your horse, you would also have a horse who was incapable of hard work.

Over time, a new movement – 'barefoot' – emerged from the US and from Europe, and its practice became notorious in the British horse world. As horse owners, we heard about the barefoot movement and both independently met people who had succumbed to this new fad.

It was presented as a 'natural' way of keeping your horse, which was understandably an extremely attractive idea to many people. Perhaps another attraction was that 'barefoot' seemed a great way of saving money, as you apparently simply took the shoes off your horse and never had to pay another farrier's bill.

Some owners of these barefoot horses explained that, as horses were not shod in the wild, it was wrong to shoe them in domestication. The problem was that although these 'barefooters' religiously kept their horses unshod, in practice they seemed seldom to ride their horses, because their horses were rarely sound. Any work they did was limited to quiet hacking on good ground, avoiding roads and stony tracks, as the horses were usually 'footy' on these surfaces. There was certainly no question of competing on these horses.

We found this early experience of barefoot very off-putting, because our horses' welfare and soundness were of paramount importance to us, and of course we wanted to be able to carry on working and competing our horses. It seemed to be clear that, in order to keep horses sound, and in hard work, one really did need shoes.

If shoes weren't the solution, what was?

The problem was that, once we realised shoes were not ideal, there were few people who had any idea that there could be a way of working horses in the UK without shoes.

We'd heard of horses working without shoes in dry climates, but the consensus was that this would be impossible in the UK, with its damp climate and high rainfall. Even worse, we lived in two of the wettest areas of the UK, on Exmoor and in North Wales (where the average annual rainfall is 180–254 cm (70–100 in).

We knew that feral horses didn't need shoes, but we had been told time and again that this was because they weren't ridden or worked on artificial surfaces. In addition, we had seen horses in the UK who were totally lame without shoes or, at best, 'footy' on challenging surfaces.

So what pushed us to find out more? Like many people, we were forced to learn more about working horses without shoes, not out of inclination, but because we had no alternative.

Each of us had horses who were shod, and who had become lame – one with suspensory ligament damage, one with severe cracks in the hoof and one with navicular syndrome. These horses – Fari, Bailey and Ghost – drove us to try barefoot; our backs were against the wall because shoes were simply not able to keep them sound.

We were extremely fortunate, though, because we also each had one horse (Felix and Jesta) with fantastic hooves: hooves which were so sound and tough that, even straight out of shoes, Felix could work happily barefoot on all surfaces. Jesta had never been shod and miraculously, both these horses could walk, trot and canter over challenging surfaces in complete comfort, despite having 'unprotected' feet.

These were the two horses who set the benchmark for healthy hooves. On the one hand, we were backed into a corner by the lameness of three of our horses, but on the other hand we were inspired by the unshod ability of the other two.

This paradox forced us to re-examine our belief system, and to challenge, question and explore just why some hooves worked so well bare while others failed miserably. What we learnt, both from our own horses and from other people who were experimenting with barefoot, was that the form, structure and internal integrity of our horses' hooves reflected their ability to function.

3

What does a healthy hoof look like?

It is perfectly possible for an unshod horse to have unhealthy hooves, but in our experience few shod hooves are totally healthy. In other words they don't meet our benchmark for healthy hooves. However, you do see good hooves in some shod horses. Our experience has shown time and time again that these horses, with good hooves, are able to work comfortably on challenging surfaces almost as soon as their shoes come off. Perhaps they never needed their shoes in the first place.

Healthy hooves are as individual as healthy horses. The shape of an Arab's hoof and a cob's hoof will never look the same; even two horses of the same breed doing the same job will have distinctly different hooves, particularly if they live under different environmental conditions. For example, a horse living and working on sand will have a more concave hoof and a less pronounced frog, which will maximise his ability to load the hoof centrally on these surfaces. By contrast, a horse who works on the road will have a less concave hoof and a more developed frog, which will minimise peripheral loading and concussion on hard surfaces.

Most horses in the UK need to be able to work on a variety of surfaces, including conformable surfaces (arenas), hard level surfaces (roads) and surfaces with limited give (tracks and fields). The hoof will constantly try to adapt to different stimuli and environmental conditions. Therefore, it is important to realise that to achieve optimum health, hooves need to be continually exposed to different environmental stimuli. You cannot expect a horse who is kept on deep shavings and works only in an arena to have hooves that are sufficiently developed to withstand the challenges of extensive roadwork.

There are, though, characteristics that the healthiest hooves have in common.

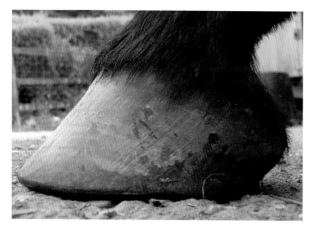

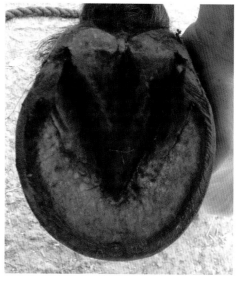

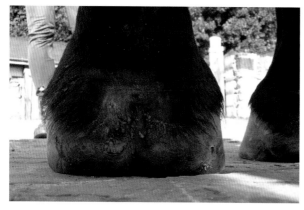

In a healthy hoof:

- The hoof wall is smooth and free from ripples.
- The frog is substantial and has a weight-bearing function.
- The digital cushion is well-developed to absorb shock.
- The hoof is loaded centrally, not peripherally.

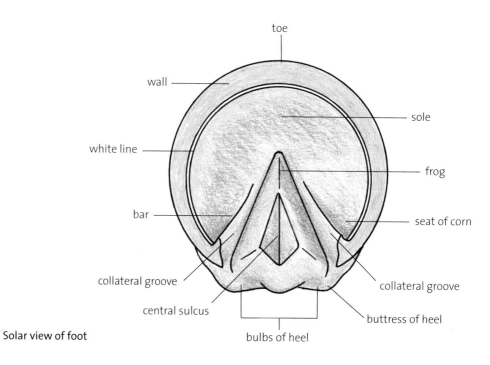

Solar view of foot

The frog

A healthy hoof will have a large, strong frog. The frog is one of the most important structures in the hoof, and is usually much more substantial in a barefoot horse than it is in a shod horse. The appearance of a truly healthy frog can surprise hoof care professionals who are used to the frogs on shod horses. So much so, in fact, that some farriery textbooks, portraying a frog that has become actively weight-bearing, describe it as over-developed.

The accompanying photos of frog prints of shod and unshod horses show clearly how much more weight and impact are taken on the frog of a barefoot horse, even on soft ground. In fact, in a healthy hoof, the frog takes a significant share, with the heels, in bearing the weight of the horse as he lands and moves on hard ground.

In a truly healthy hoof, working regularly on hard ground, if a rasp is laid across the raised hoof, the frog will be at the same level as the rasp or even appear to be proud of the heel buttresses.

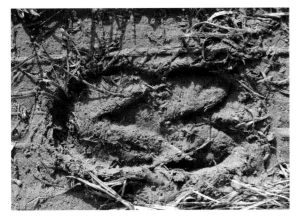

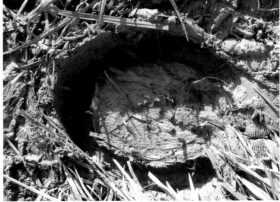

ABOVE LEFT Hoof print of a barefoot horse.

ABOVE RIGHT Hoof print of a shod horse.

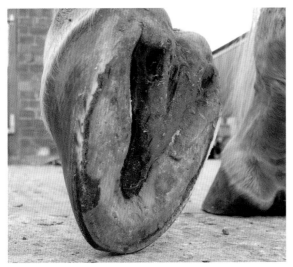

The frog is at its strongest when the horse is working on a variety of surfaces.

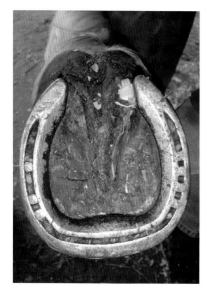

Atrophy of the frog, with resultant contraction of heels and back of foot.

As with many structures in the horse's hoof, the frog is at its strongest when the horse is working on a variety of surfaces, including abrasive and stimulating ground such as roads, gravel or stones. A barefoot horse who is not in work, or who is living and working only on soft ground like a field, arena or sandy terrain, is likely to have a less-developed frog.

Strong, healthy frogs will maintain their health and shape without needing to be cut or shaped by the farrier or trimmer. In a shod horse, pure mechanics (the rim of the shoe) mean that the frog is not able to bear as much weight, although the best shoeing will attempt to allow the frog as much stimulus as possible. Nevertheless, the combination of the added height of the shoe and the restriction of expansion and contraction caused by a shoe will normally mean that the frog is less developed. In some horses, this lack of stimulus, usually coupled with high heels, leads the frog to atrophy, with the result that the heels and the back of the foot contract.

The wall

A healthy hoof, such as in the photos at the start of this chapter, will have a smooth outer hoof wall, free from ripples (sometimes called 'growth rings') or flare (as distinct from wall deviation).

If the dorsal hoof wall begins to grow in at a changing angle (typically tighter at the coronet), this is normally a sign of an improved diet, improved circulation, or both.

So-called 'growth rings' are actually distortions in the hoof wall, which can be caused by an increase or decrease in circulation, a change in diet or a physiological event such as disease, illness or exposure to toxins. In at least one case, a horse who underwent a Hobday and tieback operation showed a dramatic 'growth ring' after the operation and grew a tighter hoof capsule at a radically improved angle, presumably owing to improved aerobic ability.

The hoof capsule on a barefoot horse who is working on varied surfaces will grow from coronet to ground in around four to six months, compared to nine to twelve months for a shod horse, or a less well-stimulated bare hoof.

Once a horse is barefoot and working hard on abrasive surfaces, the sole of the hoof receives much greater stimulus (there is simply no 'dead sole' on a hard-working barefoot horse).

In humans, stimulus to the epidermal layer of the skin on the hands and feet increases cell reproduction – this is the way in which we avoid the skin on our hands and feet from wearing away; with increased pressure the cells

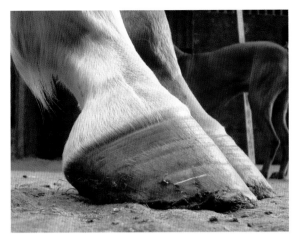 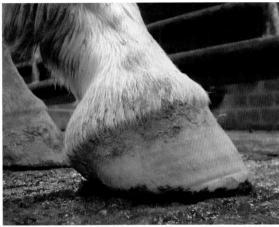

ABOVE LEFT The ring at the top of the hoof marks where the horse's shoes came off.

ABOVE RIGHT Five months later, the ring is at the bottom of the hoof and charts how quickly the hooves are growing.

multiply faster to match the increased abrasion of the skin. It has not been proved that horses have these same cells in their epidermal laminae, but it is one possible explanation of how hooves are able to respond to stimulus by growing faster. If the cells also exist in the hoof, then increased stimulus of the hooves, with more abrasive surfaces (and therefore more pressure), would prompt the epidermal laminae in the sole and hoof wall to increase cell production.

You can see the effects of this increased growth clearly in a barefoot horse who has been accustomed to doing many hours of roadwork. If the exercise regime changes, the hoof capsule will continue to grow fast enough to accommodate the original level of roadwork for some time.

One of our clients had a Warmblood mare who, for a couple of years, had been used to doing two to three hours of roadwork a day. She was then sent to stud and was no longer being exercised, but until her hooves adapted to her new lifestyle, they were growing so fast that they needed trimming every week.

The wall should be growing at a consistent angle from coronet to ground level. However, if this angle is too shallow or too steep, the result will be an imbalanced or weakened hoof. A hoof capsule unbalanced in this way will tend to over-wear at the toe or heels, resulting in a hoof which may not perform well over abrasive or uneven surfaces, whether shod or barefoot.

Generally, the hoof wall on a barefoot horse will look shorter and steeper than in a shod horse, as the distance from the coronet to the ground at the toe can be as little as 7.6 cm (3 in) or even less. It is important to emphasise, though, that we do not measure angles or toe length to use them as trimming guidelines. Differences in conformation, stance and current hoof health will result in horses needing differing dorsal wall angles and toe length.

Bruising in the hoof wall can be a sign of trauma, or even laminitis, but can also sometimes occur even in healthy hooves, without causing any problems, if the horse has worked on rough, stony ground.

Flare

Flare results from a weakness in the white line, and a lack of connection between the hoof wall and the internal structures of the hoof. Flare has been viewed in the past as a mechanical problem, caused by hoof wall growing too long (for instance at the quarters) and bowing out under the horse's weight.

In most horses, weakness in the laminar attachment of the hoof wall, which leads to stretching of the white line and flaring of the hoof wall, indicates dietary imbalance or mineral deficiencies and it is extremely unusual for flare to occur if there are no dietary problems.

Provided the hoof wall is healthily connected to the internal structures of the hoof, it will be too strong to bow out. Dissection of a healthy hoof shows it is extremely hard to detach healthy hoof wall because the laminar bond is so strong. Instead, if an otherwise healthy hoof wall is too long it will usually chip or crack off, as it grows proud of the sole.

LEFT Flare in the hoof wall.

RIGHT Stretched white line indicating flare.

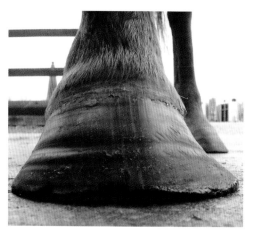
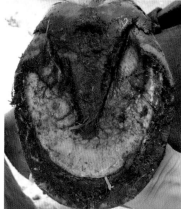

Wall deviation

Wall deviation differs from flare as it can occur even in a healthy, well-connected hoof. It reflects how the hoof is being loaded, and research shows that an external wall deviation reflects a similar variation in the pedal bone, again as a result of imbalanced loading. Sometimes this imbalance is simply a result of poor medial/lateral balance in the hoof, in which case once the hoof is centrally loaded, it will correct over a period of time.

Occasionally, the hoof is loading in an unbalanced way as a result of a conformation fault or injury elsewhere in the horse's body. If this is the case, then the wall deviation will persist as long as the fault or injury prevents the hoof from loading correctly. Wall deviation should not be mistaken for flare, as the trimming requirements for dealing with flare are completely different.

Normally, deviated hoof wall is not the strongest structure on which to support a horse's weight, but in the case in the adjacent photo, the hoof wall has had to adapt to allow the limb to receive the maximum amount of support.

This is a key practical trimming difference between flare and wall deviation – removal of flare will improve the horse's biomechanics, whereas removing a wall deviation (which is acting as a support) will normally make the horse less sound.

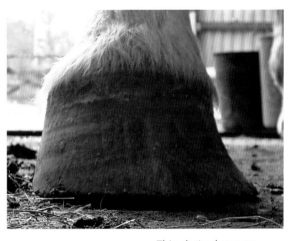

This photo shows an extreme case, where the horse has grown a medial wall deviation, which is allowing him to compensate for an old knee injury. Provided this wall deviation was respected, the horse remained sound, but the deviation was critical in allowing him to land level.

The sole

It is possible to judge the internal strength of a hoof from the depth of the collateral grooves at the back of the hoof. A strong, well-connected hoof will have deeper collateral grooves, and a sole which shows some concavity – the depth of the concavity will depend on the horse's environment. A weak hoof will have shallower collateral grooves and will look flat, or possibly even convex.

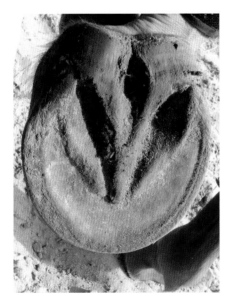

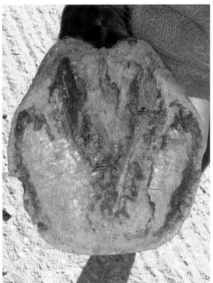

FAR LEFT Hoof showing good collateral groove depth.

LEFT Hoof showing weak collateral grooves. The heels are long and the frog weak: if the heels were to be lowered to the corresponding height of the photo on the left, the collateral groove depth would be nil.

Collateral groove depth is a more reliable indicator of hoof health than concavity alone (except in laminitic cases – See Chapter 5), because good collateral groove depth indicates a strong laminar attachment of the hoof wall to the internal structures of the hoof.

Concavity

We are used to thinking of a healthy hoof as having good concavity, but in fact the concavity of a hoof is more a function of the surfaces a horse lives on. So a horse living predominantly on flatter, harder ground will have less concavity than a horse living on sand.

A deeply concave hoof is very useful on a soft surface, but if your horse lives in an area of hard, level ground then too much concavity can actually be harmful, as the hoof will then tend to load peripherally, so horses on hard ground will generally have less solar concavity. In addition, larger hooves will appear less concave than small hooves even though both may be equally healthy. The pedal bone has roughly the same amount of concavity whether it is the bone in a Shire or a Shetland – but of course is much broader in a larger horse. The same amount of concavity looks shallower on these horses simply because it is spread over a wider area.

Surface and thickness

A healthy sole is smooth and free of cracks. Sole which flakes, chips or has black cracks is usually dead sole. This type of sole is very common in horses coming out of shoes, but once a horse is working barefoot on abrasive surfaces the sole usually abrades naturally and becomes smooth – it is almost never necessary for the sole of a barefoot horse to be trimmed by a farrier or trimmer.

The sole develops optimum thickness for the individual horse and naturally takes part of the horse's weight. This weight-bearing stimulus has been shown to be necessary in order for the pedal bone to maintain bone density. Loading the sole also allows the hoof to make maximum use of its shock-absorbing qualities.

In a healthy hoof, the sole and hoof wall are well-connected by strong epidermal laminae. On radiograph, the pedal bone will appear fairly high in the hoof capsule, with the solar corium and sole protecting it from the ground, and the lateral cartilages and digital cushion providing support in the back of the hoof.

The digital cushion

The digital cushion is the area at the back of the foot above the heel bulbs and between the lateral cartilage.

In a well-developed bare hoof the digital cushion has vertical depth and dense, tough fibro-cartilage. This provides shock absorption when the horse lands heel first at any gait. The fibro-cartilage of the digital cushion develops over a considerable period of time in response to specific stimulus, and it has 'use it or lose it' qualities.

A healthy digital cushion, when palpated, has a texture similar to dense rubber, and is enveloped by the lateral cartilages. In a strong hoof, the digital cushion fills the area between the lateral cartilages and whole area of the back of the hoof is round and full.

In a weak hoof the edges of lateral cartilages seem more pronounced, or even to be collapsing inwards, because digital cushion development is lacking. The area above the heel buttresses feels shallow and empty.

Like the frog, the digital cushion requires work on stimulating surfaces in order to function optimally. It should respond and improve fairly quickly, often strengthening within three months once shoes are removed.

As a foot becomes healthier and works harder, the overall depth of the back of the foot (from the solar surface to the top of the lateral cartilage) increases.

In a shod foot the shoe creates rigidity, which restricts hoof expansion and contraction. The shoe also reduces or, in some cases, completely re-moves the frog's load-bearing role. As the digital cushion can only develop and strengthen in response to frog pressure, both of these effects will inter-fere with the function of a healthy digital cushion. The shock-absorbing capability of the back of the foot is therefore reduced in a shod hoof.

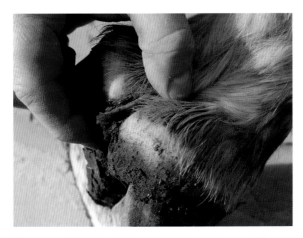

The area of digital cushion – palpating this area will reveal how developed the digital cushion is.

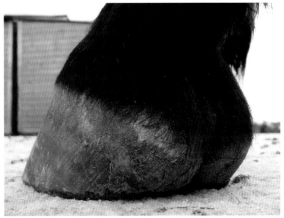

A healthy hoof showing good digital cushion development.

The artificial restriction created by the shoe can, to an extent, compensate for weakness and instability in the back of the hoof. However, it does not allow the digital cushion and lateral cartilages to improve or strengthen and therefore concussion, which would be absorbed in a healthy digital cushion, will be transmitted to other tissues in the limb which are not designed to absorb shock as efficiently.

It is possible to develop the digital cushion and to improve the function of the back of the foot, provided the horse has developed the basic internal

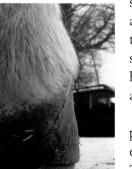

structure to his hoof. However, if a horse is shod at a very young age, the development of the internal structures of the hoof (which take around seven years to fully mature) is arrested. Such hooves are immature, and inherently unstable, and so may never regain full health and function.

It is often claimed that Thoroughbreds have poor feet, but it is possible that this is more an effect of early shoeing, which is done to many Thoroughbreds and which prevents development of the back of the foot.

A poorly developed digital cushion.

The bars

The bars appear in the back third of the solar surface of the foot as an extension of the hoof wall. Healthy hooves vary more in their bars than in any other structure. Some horses grow long bars; others grow very little. Often, in a healthy foot, bars are fairly straight and parallel to the line of

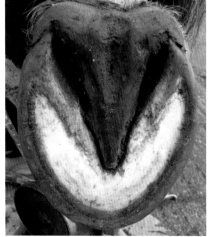

the frog; in an unhealthy, contracted hoof they will be curved, almost in a pincer shape, but over time will straighten as the hoof de-contracts.

In a healthy hoof, which is exercising over adequate mileage and receiving stimulus on abrasive terrain, the bars usually maintain themselves and do not benefit from aggressive trimming.

The white line

The white line is a zone between the junction of the inner and outer structures of the hoof. Anatomically, this is where the epidermal laminae are visible, bonding the sensitive internal structures and the hoof wall together. A healthy bare foot will have a narrow white line, which will be barely visible except as a change in texture between the sole and hoof wall.

A hoof with healthy bars, also showing a well-connected white line.

The white line is often the first part of the hoof to show damage, and appears to stretch, becoming wider once the laminar attachment between the epidermal laminae and the hoof wall is compromised.

A stretched white line (as shown in the photo on page 28) is normally the result of dietary or metabolic problems, and will be exacerbated by mech-anical forces (i.e. the weight of the horse). The outcome is that the white line loses attachment and in all cases the dorsal hoof wall will distort to a greater or lesser extent.

A stretched white line has microscopic gaps which can be entry points for bacterial and fungal infections. These can attack the sensitive structures of the hoof, and this is one of the reasons why a laminitic horse is more prone to hoof abscesses.

Once an area of laminae has been damaged, it cannot repair, and the stretched white line will remain until new laminae have been produced and stronger, well-connected hoof wall has grown down. This will be visible from the angle of the dorsal hoof wall at the coronet. A stretched white line, is a vulnerable area which can trap gravel or small stones, but these problems are an effect of the stretch rather than a cause.

The heels

The heels on a well-developed bare hoof will appear low when the foot is picked up, as there will be very little wall height above the sole. When viewed from the side, however, the development in the back of the foot will cause the hoof to look as if it has plenty of heel height; the strong digital cushion means that there is great depth from the solar surface (where the heels meet the ground) to the top of the lateral cartilage.

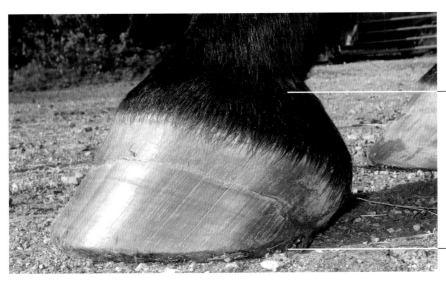

A hoof showing strong heel depth.

— top of lateral cartilage

— depth from solar surface

A shod foot viewed from the side will also look as if it has plenty of heel height, and the hoof will be further raised by the shoe. In contrast to a bare hoof, however, this height will be constituted by hoof wall which is proud of the sole at the heel buttresses. The shoe tends to prevent or minimise the development of the digital cushion, particularly if the frog is weak, and in these cases, high hoof wall takes the place of developed internal structure.

The hoof, even when shed, is dynamic and will try to compensate with higher heels for structures that are deficient elsewhere. If the digital cushion and frog weaken sufficiently, the back of the foot can even ossify (the lateral cartilages become calcified and rigid as in sidebone), perhaps in an attempt to stabilise the area.

If the back of the foot is compromised, particularly in a horse who has been poorly shod, it can lead to heels becoming collapsed or under-run. It is also common in a shod foot for the frog to prolapse and this, together with the under-run heels, can make heels look long when viewed from the side, although they are short when viewed from the sole.

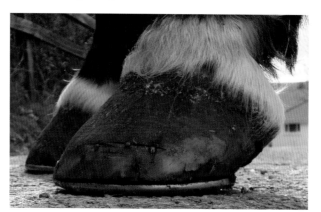

High heels but poor development of internal structure.

Fortunately, once a horse starts to land heel first out of shoes, the strength and depth of the back of the foot – particularly the digital cushion and frog – usually improves rapidly and then provides support to the heels internally.

Weight-bearing properties

Where a horse is shod, the shoe and the hoof wall become the primary weight-bearing structure. The frog has a more limited role when the majority of the horse's weight is peripherally loaded in this way. (See photos on page 25 for a clear indication of this.) Research has shown that this peripheral loading places stresses on the internal structures of the hoof, and we will look at this in more detail in Chapter 4, How Do Hooves Work?

Where a horse is barefoot with a healthy hoof, more of his weight is centrally loaded, and many structures have an active weight-bearing role; the heel (including the digital cushion), frog, inner hoof wall and the sole all helping to support the weight of the horse together. As these areas all bear weight, they are also all stimulated, which we believe is essential to the long-term health of the hoof.

The hoof/pastern angle

Traditionally, a straight hoof/pastern angle has been viewed as a benchmark of healthy hooves, and some farriery textbooks have recommended trimming or shoeing a hoof using hoof/pastern angle (from the dorsal wall to the fetlock) as one of the main external guidelines.

It is undoubtedly true that a sound, healthy hoof will have a 'correct' hoof/pastern angle, but we find that using it as a guideline for trimming or shoeing tends to be a case of putting the cart before the horse. There are two main reasons for this.

First, the way the horse is standing and loading his hooves constantly changes as his weight shifts, and this will significantly affect hoof/pastern angle, and so the angle will often be too dynamic or changeable to be a useful guideline over time.

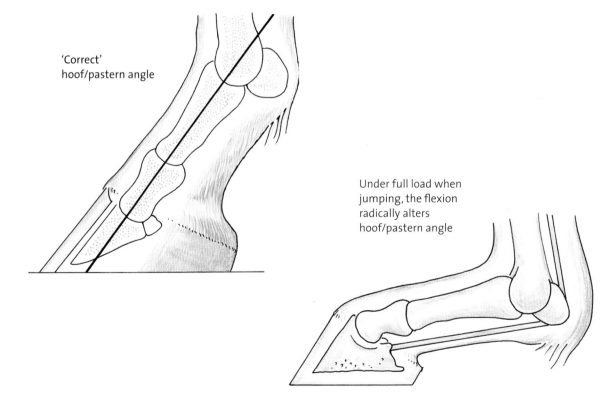

'Correct' hoof/pastern angle

Under full load when jumping, the flexion radically alters hoof/pastern angle

Second, and more importantly, an incorrect hoof/pastern angle is always a symptom of a weakness elsewhere in the foot. This can be a problem in the back of the hoof – such as a poorly developed digital cushion – or a weakness in the attachment of the hoof wall to the internal structures that may have led to a long toe or under-run heel.

It is possible with shoeing to 'correct' the hoof/pastern angle, but the danger is that the external appearance of the hoof capsule (the dorsal wall angle) is improved without dealing with the underlying weakness. In this scenario, correcting the angle without improving the overall integrity of the hoof means that the hoof is liable to continue to run forward, constantly losing correct hoof/pastern angle, and over time will seriously deteriorate. We believe this is a consequence of the stress caused by peripherally loading a hoof that has weak internal structures.

Our preference is to try to rehabilitate the whole hoof structure, rather than focusing on improving a single (though important) angle. Once a hoof has developed optimum health, with a strong digital cushion, well-developed lateral cartilages and tight connection of the laminae, the hoof capsule will be sufficiently strong to maintain the correct hoof/pastern angle.

Internal strength is therefore the foundation upon which correctly functioning hooves are built.

Self-maintenance

One of the recurring features of the healthiest hooves is the fact that they need little or no intervention in the form of trimming.

The healthiest hoof is one which is working hard, covering high mileage on challenging surfaces and receiving constant stimulus. The ideal hoof will develop and wear in a way which supports the horse's own movement and conformation, and as a result will be naturally balanced for that horse.

In this perfect scenario, the hoof will maintain itself, and it is only if his diet or environment changes, or if the horse has a more serious conformation abnormality or has been injured, that the hoof may be unable to maintain itself.

In reality, a self-maintaining, perfectly balanced hoof is hard to achieve in a domestic situation, but it remains the ideal from the horse's point of view.

4

How do hooves work?

In all natural action the heels come to the ground first, not the toe…the heels are the part to receive the shock and in doing this the frog or foot pad plays a very prominent part.

Professor W. Jones Anstey FWCF, FZS, *The Care of the Horse*, 1929

As long ago as 1929 there was a basic understanding of the importance of correct hoof function. Understanding how hooves work when at their optimum is essential if we are to develop awareness of their fragility when function is restricted. Without correct function, a hoof's structure and performance will be ultimately compromised.

Over the years, many theories on improving hoof function have been developed and discussed. Most, however, have concentrated on looking at how hooves function with metal shoes, almost as if it would be unthinkable to assess bare hooves.

Perhaps this is because the traditional belief is that hooves are unable to function without metal shoes under the loads and stresses associated with everyday riding, competition or driving. It also reveals the massive contradiction of thought in the 'conventional world', where a hoof is considered robust enough to have nails driven into it and red-hot metal burnt onto it, yet so delicate and fragile that even in an arena it needs a rim of metal for support and protection.

This set of beliefs is one major reason for the shortage of research on the function of fully developed healthy hooves. There is another, very pragmatic reason for this shortage.

Studying healthy hooves requires a supply of cadavers that have been obtained from horses on an optimum diet, in an optimum environment, exercising over an optimum distance on challenging surfaces, every day since birth.

Hooves of this kind are extremely unusual in a domestic setting and it is even more unlikely that you will find healthy, hard-working hooves on the bench of a research scientist. Why? Because horses with such hooves are likely to remain sound for so many years that the trip to the abattoir, or gift to the research centre, just never becomes an option.

So what material does tend to end up in today's research centre? Mostly it is horses who have been put down because of unsolvable health problems, frequently involving the hoof or lower limb.

So herein lies a problem: if researchers tend only to dissect or analyse unhealthy hooves, then how do we know how a truly healthy hoof functions?

The latest research

The answer lies in research that has been stimulated and fuelled by the 'barefoot movement' and studies into the feral horses in the US. Observations by Gene Ovnicek, Registered Master Farrier (US) and developer of Natural Balance shoeing, and ongoing research by Dr Robert Bowker, VMD PhD, Professor at Michigan State University Veterinary Medical Centre have revealed vast differences between how healthy hooves actually function compared to what was traditionally thought.

Depression theory

Traditionally there have been many theories surrounding hoof function. For many years it was proposed that, as the hoof depressed on contact with the ground, the frog acted as a 'pump' and, when hitting a surface, would squash, circulate blood around the foot and provide shock-absorption. The long-held view was that as long as a shoe did not restrict the back third of the foot this 'pump' would still function. Therefore nails in horseshoes were not placed in the back third of the hoof wall. This theory has now been shown to be incorrect and this is why even without nails in the back third a shod hoof experiences restriction of blood flow, flexion and reduced shock-absorbing function.

Pressure theory

A recent experiment conducted by Dr Robert Bowker of Michigan State University found that, in an anaesthetised horse, when a pressure probe was inserted into the digital cushion, negative pressure was evident when the hoof was under load. Once the hoof was unloaded the pressure reading returned to zero. It is unclear, however, whether the same readings would be gained when a horse was in locomotion. Certainly the action of loading appears to be part of a complicated hymadynamic process where blood is moved through the hoof and all its structures. This it is far from the traditional view of the hoof operating as a basic pump, which held that blood was simply pushed out of the hoof in the loading phase. Perhaps imagining the hoof as a water-filled balloon helps us to understand how blood is moved through its structures. If you press on the water-filled balloon with your hand to simulate a hoof in movement, rolling from the back forward to the point of breakover, then you will find that the water dissipates forwards, to the side and then to the back. If Dr Bowker's experiments are correct, the pressure as this happens at impact in a moving hoof could be quite considerable: 20-40 kilo Pascals, which approximates to 1.35–2.7 kg per 6.5 square cm (3–6 lb per square in). This indicates the possibility that a very effective hydraulic system is in operation in a correctly functioning healthy hoof. Crucially, even when the experts cannot agree on exactly *how* the venous system of the hoof functions, they agree that, in a healthy hoof, the blood flow through the venous plexus creates a dampening effect which has an important role in reducing concussion as the hoof lands on the ground.

Energy dissipation

At the same time, venous blood is perfused or 'squished' through a massive network of capillaries that are part of the venous system. These capillaries are like very thin straws and in a healthy hoof there is a multitude of them. This creates a myriad of channels for the blood to be forced through and thus dissipates energy. Think of the force of water at high pressure in a hosepipe and how strong it can be. If you want to dissipate the water's energy then you allow the water to flow through many small holes, as in a watering rose. The resistance created by the small holes means energy is

Blood capillaries

the capillaries are like very skinny straws

a myriad of capillaries connect to the veins

dissipated and the flow loses its force and can sprinkle over plants without harming them. The more holes, the more resistance, the more energy is dissipated.

Hydraulic shock-absorption

A healthy hoof will be rich in this myriad of veins and capillaries, creating perfusion which absorbs shock hydraulically, preventing high-frequency energy from damaging tendons, ligaments or bone. In an unhealthy hoof, which has poorly developed structures owing to peripheral loading (as with a shoe), this system of irrigating the blood through the hoof may be either impaired or even simply absent. This means that the blood races through the hoof without slowing, energy is not dissipated as efficiently and, over time, injury will occur.

Dr Bowker has also shown that the solar corium, which lies between the pedal bone and the sole, contains a high proportion of proteoglycans, which give it a gel-like consistency. He theorises that this provides a shock-absorbing cushion which helps dissipate energy as the hoof lands. Again, when a hoof is peripherally loaded, much of the benefit is lost, but once the hoof is centrally loaded, the sole is able to thicken and build in depth and can become strong enough to traverse challenging surfaces without bruising.

Heel-first landing

It is widely agreed that horses, like humans, need to land heel first. A healthy hoof will engage the whole shock-absorption system by engaging he back third of the hoof with the ground in a heel-first landing (see Jacket photo). The shock-absorption system is located externally at the heel buttresses, the frog and the bars, and internally at the frog corium, digital cushion and lateral cartilages. In a healthy hoof these structures work intricately and in conjunction with each other. When the shock-absorption system is weak, under-developed or deformed, then the way blood is moved around the hoof and energy dissipated is compromised.

It seems, then, that optimal hoof function revolves around the development of strong and healthy structures, particularly in the back of the foot.

Flexion and stimulus

The whole hoof needs to flex in a multitude of directions if it is to develop strength and build itself into a fully functioning, effective shock-absorbing structure. The more it is used, the better it develops. All structures of the hoof, both internal and external, rely on stimulation of movement over varied surfaces to form properly. Without stimulus and flexion, hooves have no other choice than to compensate for lack of development.

Under-developed, peripherally loaded hooves generally have a brittle pedal bone, thin solar corium, thin hoof walls, thin lateral cartilages, soft digital cushion and weak, long laminae. Developed hooves generally have a dense pedal bone and thick corium, particularly in the outer periphery just where load-bearing and expansion are both needed and received. They have thick hoof walls, thick lateral cartilages, a firm and fibrous digital cushion and strong, short laminae.

There is no doubt that all hooves, whether healthy or not, dissipate energy, but those which have strong developed structures working together in concert are the ones likely to protect the limb above and remain free from injury.

Differences observed in foals

Domestic foals

Gene Ovnicek has highlighted how, sadly, from the very first days of a domestic horse's life, his lifestyle and environment conspire to prevent structures developing correctly.

Typically, domestic foals are kept in contained and restricted environments. Turning them out in a field with soft footing is just not enough to generate the 'going to the gym and working out' environment which will stimulate, strengthen and develop the internal hoof structures enough to provide a strong foundation for the huge weight of horse they will carry as an adult.

Think of the hoof as being just like any other part of the horse's body that needs developing. A Grand Prix dressage horse takes years of correct exercise to develop the body muscle strength to allow him to carry himself … hooves should be no different.

Feral foals

Dr Bowker has noted that the hooves of a foal go through some very remarkable changes in the first few weeks of life if allowed access to maximum movement over abrasive terrain. At birth, the fore and hind hooves are identical in shape but within two weeks the fore hooves have become rounder. In addition, the heels wear level with the frog, allowing this structure to become tough and broad, thus providing the role of supporting the bony column while the digital cushion develops.

This foal is on soft grass: foals' feet change markedly in the first weeks of life if they move freely over abrasive terrain.

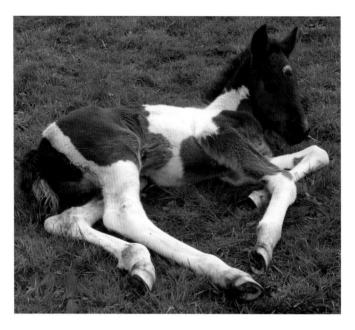

Proprioception

Nerve endings in the human foot constantly send messages to our brain, giving us feedback on where, and on what surfaces, we are standing and moving over. This neural information, called proprioception, enables us to constantly adjust our muscles, tendons and ligaments, allowing us to balance in response to changing terrain and speed.

Research[1] has shown that when the human foot is encased in even a soft, supportive running shoe, proprioception is impaired and the risk of both acute (sudden, accidental) and chronic (long term) injury substantially increases. Conversely, the researchers[2] found that barefoot runners suffer a much lower incidence of injury. The researchers attribute this to improved proprioception, and the fact that barefoot runners, unlike those running in shoes, are able to alter their behaviour to reduce shock in response to impact force. The same researchers later concluded:

> The modern running shoe, and footwear in general, have successfully diminished sensory feedback without diminishing the injury-inducing impact, a dangerous situation.[3]

It is also suggested that the sensory feedback provided by bare feet in humans is likely to improve balance.[4]

Interestingly, research in humans has shown that the shock absorption provided by 'cushioned' running shoes is in fact illusory.[5] Even when heel cushioning was increased in shoes, the impact forces on the limb remained the same. The problem is that, with more cushioning, it *feels* as if we are better protected, so we fail to compensate as much for the increased force.[6] This 'false sense of security', it is proposed, may contribute to the higher risk of injury when wearing shoes.[7]

A friend of ours who started running barefoot hadn't realised just how much his proprioception had been compromised in trainers. He had previously often found running over uneven ground difficult, resulting in his feet slipping and his ankles twisting. However, he noticed that, even the first time he ran without shoes, he seemed to sense the ground and compensate for his footing much more effectively. He now seldom slips and has not twisted an ankle since. Just how quickly his proprioception kicked in surprised him, but it was also surprising to find that he adapted to being able to run along tarmac comfortably in less than a month.

Another fascinating aspect was that, running in trainers, he usually came back with a sore hip, and was in fact being treated by an osteopath for this very problem. Running barefoot, he noticed that he shortened his stride on hard surfaces– something he failed to do in shoes – and that this adaptive response reduced the impact on his hip. It no longer hurt when he came back from a run.

If we humans, with our very static feet, are better able to load, absorb shock and balance without shoes, then how much more efficiently can horses compensate with dynamic, bare hooves? Add to this the fact that running shoes are causing, rather than solving, problems for us, despite being soft, flexible and padded – and you have to wonder about the effect of a rigid, metal shoe on a horse's hoof.

Although equivalent research has not been carried out on the horse, it is reasonable to conclude that a nailed-on, metal shoe will also limit proprioception and shock-absorption in the horse in a similar way. We have certainly observed frequently horses who seem more confident on their feet, and less prone to tripping, over-reaching, and strain once they are out of shoes.

Similarly, we have frequently seen that a horse recently out of shoes, who still has to develop strong digital cushions, will tend to shorten his stride slightly when moving from a grass verge on to a road in trot. By comparison, a shod horse trotting alongside will not seem to notice that the surface has changed.

Perhaps, rather than being a sign of foot pain (as some riders would assume), this is in fact a sign that the unshod horse is aware of the increased concussion and is protecting his joints.

Certainly, once horses are barefoot with strong, shock-absorbing digital cushions, they seem more than happy to extend their stride even on hard surfaces.

The horse's feet as neuro-sensory organs

Treating horses' hooves differently from other animals' feet has perhaps dulled our ability to see them as a sensory area, able to detect the environment. The hard, keratinised outer wall of the horse's hoof is akin to a human nail. No one would disagree that Mother Nature has designed human nails essentially as protective structures (which some people like to decorate!). Human nails are designed to carry minimal load and are stronger when they are short. Why shouldn't a horse's hoof wall have evolved to be the same?

On our hands the most sensitive area for detecting the environment is at our fingertips. Similarly, the sole, frog and heel bulb areas of a horse's hoof have also been shown to contain two types of neuro-sensory cells.

Pacinian corpuscles are neuro-sensory cells that are sensitive to deep-pressure touch and high-frequency gross pressure changes. They are found in the bulbs of the heel which, in a well-developed, hard-working barefoot horse, will be engaged with the ground as the horse correctly lands heel first. These cells only 'fire' when the horse is moving. Meissner corpuscles are located in areas of the human body where light touch and sensitivity is required. (These are the same cells we have in our fingertips and they enable us to feel our world in a highly complex way.) In the horse they are located in the frog, suggesting that this structure needs to be in contact with the ground in order to provide crucial feedback to the horse.

One of our clients noticed how her horse, when shod, would pull back on his lead rope until it broke if he happened to stand on it. Once unshod, when the same thing happened, the horse still pulled back but, when he felt the resistance, he connected this with having stood on the rope and merely stepped off without breaking it.

In a more dramatic example, co-author Nic came off one of her barefoot horses out hunting, and to the horror of a watching rider, the horse appeared to trample on her. Sure enough, when Nic took her coat off, she found hoof prints up the back, but she had not even been bruised. She believes the horse felt what he was treading on and kindly shifted his weight to avoid injuring her!

Moving straight...

Very few, if any, humans move on a completely straight track, and successful human runners will usually pronate to some extent. Pronation is when the outside edge of the heel strikes the ground first and then the foot rolls inwards, and a moderate pronation is not only normal but required for efficient movement and shock absorption.

In the same way, many sound, hard-working horses will breakover slightly off centre, with the foot 'rolling' inwards or outwards (the equivalent of pronation in humans).

Horses with perfectly straight limbs will breakover at the toe, but horses with less than perfect forelimb conformation may breakover off centre. Most horses will nevertheless load both medial and lateral aspects of the forefeet evenly, despite their breakover being slightly off centre. A metal shoe, particularly with a toe clip, can interfere with where this breakover occurs. If the horse cannot dictate breakover then, over time, as the horse repeats his steps thousand and thousands of time, the loading of the limb above will be incorrect for that horse and injury may occur.

It is common for horses to load their hind feet very slightly to the lateral side first, owing to the different action of the hind limbs, but this is not visible to the naked eye, and can only be seen on high resolution, slow motion footage of the horse moving. In rare cases, however, the reason the horse is loading unevenly is nothing to do with the hoof, but arises as compensation for the horse's conformation, an old injury, weakness or discomfort elsewhere in the body.

Horses have a much better ability than humans to compensate for such things as conformation – unlike our feet, their hooves are dynamic, and are constantly adapting to the loading of the limbs above them.

If you watch the top competitors running in a marathon, you will see that no two people move the same way, and that few if any of them will move straight – and yet most will be 'sound' and perfectly able to complete the marathon in their target time. Notwithstanding this, we naturally tend to believe that horses should move perfectly straight (although we are not capable of this ourselves!) and we often try, through shoeing, to impose straightness upon them, in the belief that a rim of metal can relieve strain elsewhere.

However, research in human athletes has shown that attempts to correct pronation are usually doomed to failure, and that, in fact, the type of shoe worn does not significantly affect movement – although there is a measurable difference between being barefoot and wearing shoes.[8] In fact the wearers of expensive shoes that were supposed to stop over-pronation experienced a much higher rate of injury than those in cheap shoes, and barefoot runners had the lowest injury rates of all.[9]

Compensation

Comparing the anatomical structure between unhealthy and healthy hooves has highlighted the way our domestic horses are frequently compensating for failed internal structure and lack of neural feedback. A toe-first landing may occur mechanically as a consequence of a long hoof, but it may also be a way of compensating for weak structures that are causing caudal heel pain.

Many shod horses will be most reluctant to move along the uneven verges of a road at speed. They will compensate by choosing the smoothness of the road, even though it involves more concussion, perhaps because lack of proprioception and neural feedback makes the verge feel an unsafe place to be.

In the UK, hundreds of dissections of domestic hooves have revealed a huge variation in the development of all aspects of hoof structure from lateral cartilage to wall, from sole to digital cushion. The majority of these hooves have been shod for many years: for years peripheral loading has been the ultimate compensation for hooves that are far from healthy.

Comparing healthy and unhealthy structures

Digital cushion

The digital cushion sits at the back of the foot directly under the frog and plays a huge role in the ability of the horse to absorb shock effectively.

This vascularised, well-developed digital cushion is very rare in the hooves of domestic horses. When a foal is born, the digital cushion is made up of a fatty, fibrous tissue, hyaline cartilage, which needs to develop through pressure and release impact. This impact will only occur if the frog is in contact with the ground and the hoof experiences miles and miles of movement over challenging surfaces. Cells called proteoglycans need to be stimulated by movement to turn the hyaline cartilage into fibrous cartilage.

A healthy digital cushion is white in colour, with tough cartilaginous material running through it (see right-hand photo page 55). In a healthy hoof at least a third of the back of the foot becomes fibro-cartilage and biomechanically this is the best material to have in the back of the hoof for strength and shock absorption. As a consequence, in a healthy hoof there will be a ratio of 2:1 or less between the length of the pedal bone and the distance from the end of the pedal bone to the back of the heel.

By contrast, in a poorly developed hoof, the ratio between the pedal bone and the area occupied by the digital cushion can be as high as 3:1. In its undeveloped state the digital cushion will be lacking vascularisation, and be soft, yellow and fatty. This fatty consistency is just not robust enough to act as a shock-absorber underneath the pedal bone and the bony column above.

The force created as the horse's foot lands demands a thick, fibrous digital cushion, yet in the hundreds of dissections performed in the UK less than 0.2 per cent of horses have had this type of fully developed digital cushion.

Section through centre of foot and lower limb

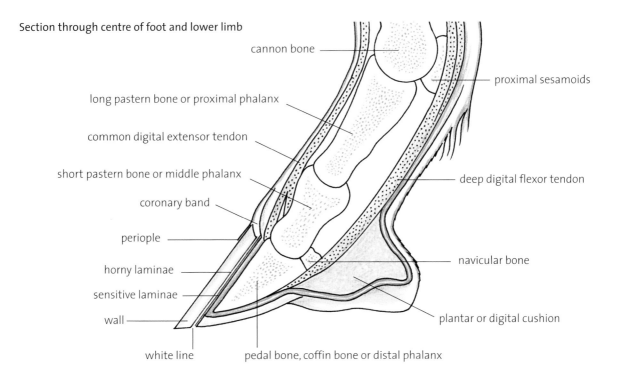

cannon bone

proximal sesamoids

long pastern bone or proximal phalanx

common digital extensor tendon

short pastern bone or middle phalanx

deep digital flexor tendon

coronary band

periople

horny laminae

navicular bone

sensitive laminae

wall

plantar or digital cushion

white line

pedal bone, coffin bone or distal phalanx

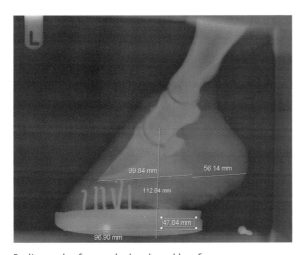

Radiograph of a poorly developed hoof.

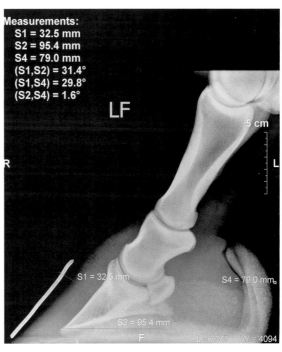

Measurements:
S1 = 32.5 mm
S2 = 95.4 mm
S4 = 79.0 mm
(S1,S2) = 31.4°
(S1,S4) = 29.8°
(S2,S4) = 1.6°

Radiograph showing healthy ratio of pedal bone and the area occupied by the digital cushion. This horse had been diagnosed with navicular syndrome six years earlier, but had subsequently spent five years barefoot.

Rehabilitation of domestic horses with severely compromised hooves has shown that the digital cushion can develop in all ages of horse. Even the most retarded of digital cushions, given a sympathetic environment, the correct engagement and time, can make some sort of recovery and regain a degree if not all their function.

For example the adjacent radiograph showing a very healthy ratio of nearly 1:1 was taken of a nineteen-year-old horse. He had been lame, and was diagnosed with navicular six years earlier, but has been barefoot and sound for five years. He came out of bar shoes with a weak, underdeveloped digital cushion, but despite his age was able to develop a much stronger back of the foot with correct environment and work.

Lateral cartilage

Lateral cartilages are attached to the upper sides of the pedal bone and although little research exists about their proper function, our experience with healthy hooves has shown that they play a major role in supporting the return venous blood flow, aiding in the dissipation of energy and shock absorption in the back third of the hoof.

Cartilage in other parts of the body does not have blood supply, yet healthy lateral cartilage is unique in having a group of veins actually running through it. Blood flowing through these veins comes from the solar venous plexus, the group of tiny veins covering the sole. This plays a key role in absorbing impact and dissipating energy.

Lateral cartilage should be highly vascularised, flexible and at least 0.6 mm ($^{24}/_{1,000}$ in) thick, yet dissections in the UK show again and again thin cartilage, often less than 0.2 mm ($^{8}/_{1,000}$ in) thick, with blood routes which are either poorly developed or non-existent. In healthy hooves you will find 20 to 30 vascular chambers; capillaries which travel physically through and around the outside of these structures. In the under-developed hooves we typically have for dissection you will be lucky to see even one!

BELOW LEFT A vascularised lateral cartilage.

BELOW RIGHT An unvascularised lateral cartilage.

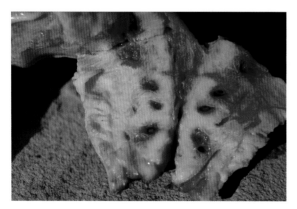

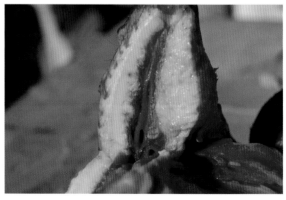

Dr Bowker has shown that these vascular chambers are aiding energy dissipation. When they are absent it stands to reason that the lateral cartilages will not be dissipating energy efficiently so that energy will be transferred to other structures.

Unhealthy lateral cartilages are thinner, offering less support to the back third of the hoof. A foot that is 11–12 cm (approx. 4½ in) wide where the lateral cartilages have combined width of 0.4 cm (⅙ in) is not going to be as strong as one where the cartilages have a combined width of 1.2 cm (just under ½ in). In a healthy hoof, the lateral cartilages will be three to four times thicker, so providing a massive superstructure for palmar support. In the unhealthy hoof the percentage of palmar tissue is so low that the load shifts forward to the pedal bone, relocating a considerable load onto ligaments and other structures.

Lateral cartilages are directly above the bars and, in a foal's immature hooves, their development starts from stimulus to the bar area. Dissection on very healthy hooves suggests that the development spreads outwards to form a strong bridge-like structure, which melds with the digital cushion. This type of structure is never seen in hooves that have been peripherally loaded for long periods of time and therefore not engaged correctly.

Lack of vascularisation in a lateral cartilage can lead to ossification (known as sidebone). This ossification further prevents flexion of the whole hoof structure, so contributing to an unhealthy spiral. In some horses, the hooves have become so debilitated that sidebone becomes a compensatory structure. The rigidity allows their hooves some function even though they are severely compromised.

Sole

The sole consists of horn produced from solar papillae, tiny finger-like structures attached to the base of the pedal bone. It is formed in platelets that overlap each other. Observation has suggested that the bars also have a role in forming sole, as some solar tissue seems to migrate forward from this area.

A healthy sole will be up to 2 cm (¾ in) thick, densely compact and resistant to pressure. The sole's ability to compress to become a dense and tough material has been much underestimated; so too has its ability to respond to wear stimulus and increase the speed of growth to match wear.

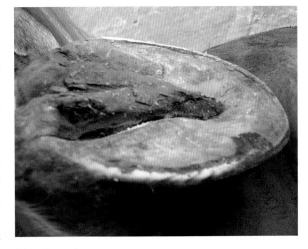

A healthy sole.

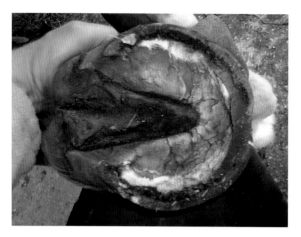

A poor sole.

An interesting comparison is with the skin on the fingertips of rock-climbers. Although this skin is rapidly abraded while climbing, rock-climbers' fingertips heal extremely quickly. This is likely to be because the considerable stimulus and abrasion their fingertips receive while climbing results in both skin growth and repair being accelerated. In our experience the sole of the horse's hoof appears to respond in the same way.

A weak sole will often present itself as being thin and flexible to thumb pressure. Studies in the UK have revealed a huge number of domestic horses exhibiting what we believe to be compression of the solar corium. This compression produces dark areas of degraded sub-solar tissue, which represent poor attachment when seen under microscopic observation. We theorise that this is the result of the sole being crushed and starved of nutrients.

Laminae

Dermal laminae grow on the outer face of the pedal bone and interlace with the epidermal laminae on the inside of the hoof wall. Together they attach the hoof wall to the bone.

Studies on hooves have shown that there are physically fewer laminae in the healthy hoof of a horse who has lived on challenging surfaces on an appropriate diet. Laminae in healthy hooves are short, chunky and fat. These thick and substantial laminae produce a hoof capsule capable of supporting greater weight and dealing with greater forces.

Conversely, horses who have long toes and flared hoof walls produce laminae that are thinner, longer and much closer together. Observations have shown that these types of weak hooves have a greater density of laminae, which is a weakening situation. These hooves are unlikely to be able to support the weight of the horse. The forces exerted in the hoof during loading and breakover are likely to stretch and bend these weak laminae. Dr Bowker has observed that laminae under stress, often at the toe or where the hoof is flared, split or 'bifurcate', becoming thinner and longer. This process affects blood flow because there is the same amount of blood but an increased surface area to keep healthy.

Bifurcation is part of the natural system of increasing the width of the hoof from foal to adult. It happens naturally in the foal as a result of growth and movement, but in the adult horse it seems to occur as an adaptive response to stress in the hoof and, unlike bifurcation in the foal, is not beneficial.

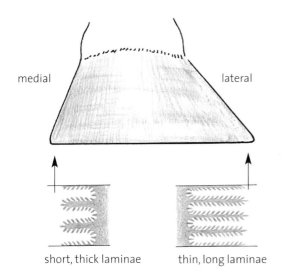

The process of bifurcation

medial

lateral

short, thick laminae   thin, long laminae

Imbalanced/assymetrical hooves
and how laminae bifurcate as a
result of stress

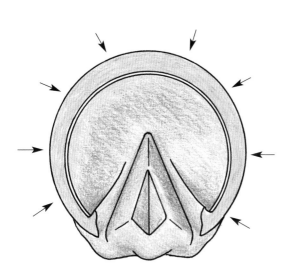

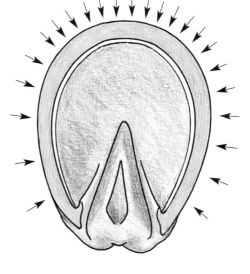

HEALTHY HOOF

UNHEALTHY HOOF

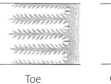

Toe   Quarters

Toe   Quarters

The arrows show how the laminae bifurcate
and become thinner, longer, weaker and more
numerous when the hoof is put under the
stress of peripheral loading

When a hoof is peripherally loaded, the hoof wall, which is not a primary loading structure, is placed under stress, therefore the laminae are more likely to bifurcate and the hoof to flare. This type of flaring indicates loss of laminar attachment and goes hand-in-hand with sole sensitivity. Loss of laminar attachment creates flat feet and a stretched white line susceptible to bacterial and fungal invasion. A horse on an optimum diet, receiving optimum exercise on a variety of challenging surfaces, will never develop this type of flare.

Hoof wall

Traditionally, it was believed that the hoof wall was generated purely from the coronary band. However when you look at a foal's foot, the shape is an inverted cone (see photo page 63), with the wall at ground level being narrower than the wall at the coronet. In an adult horse, a healthy hoof is the shape of a cone that develops naturally as the horse matures, there being a 20 per cent increase in area from coronet to ground.

If the traditional theory was correct, then it would be impossible to generate this cone shape. It seems likely, then, that the laminae must be responsible not only for attachment but also for the generation of additional hoof wall as the hoof grows down the capsule.

Observation proves that a substantial amount of wall material is produced as the hoof grows down, which cannot have been formed from the coronet. Dr Bowker's recent research has proved that up to 30 per cent of the hoof wall is produced internally, from the epidermal laminae, allowing the hoof wall to thicken as it grows down the capsule. This enables hooves to develop a cone shape, repair themselves as they grow, and mend cracks and defects in the hoof wall from internally.

By contrast, it is interesting to note that some horses seem never to develop healthy, cone-shaped hooves but have narrow, boxy, foal-shaped hooves even into adulthood. Very often these hooves are seen in horses who have been stabled for the majority of their time as adult horses, and it would be interesting to discover whether the lack of movement suffered by these horses has caused less bifurcation of laminae, and hence restricted the natural process of the hoof wall thickening as the horse matures.

The thicker the hoof wall the better, as the hoof wall's primary purpose is to provide a protective surface over the hoof's internal structures. A dorsal wall thickness of over 3 cm (1⅕ in) has been observed through digital radiography on healthily hooved horses, but in weak hooves it can be less than half of that.

A healthy hoof wall has the same ability to respond to stimulus and increase the speed of growth to match wear, as does the sole. In a hard-working bare foot the hoof wall will often travel from coronet to ground in less than five months. This adaptive acceleration in growth enables the hoof to withstand many miles over challenging surfaces.

In contrast, a hoof that has been peripherally loaded over a long period of time will not have had the stimulus needed to promote thick, strong or fast growth. The wall of a shod hoof is generally recognised to take at least nine months to grow from coronet to ground and possibly even twelve months.

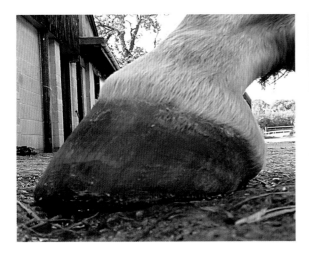
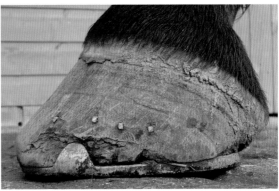

LEFT A strong hoof wall.

ABOVE A crumbly hoof wall.

Slow growth can appear hand-in-hand with a weak, crumbly wall that will be vulnerable to cracking when subjected to nailing. Interestingly, once the peripheral loading is replaced by central loading there will frequently be a very strong horizontal line that demarcates the point at which the shoes were removed and the diet improved. This line often shows a thicker wall, maybe 2 mm (1/12 in) or even 4 mm (1/6 in) thicker, travelling down the wall. Even though we have seen this many, many times we still marvel at the ability of the hoof to repair and regenerate itself when exposed to the correct kind of stimulus and diet.

Frog

A healthy frog engaged on a challenging surface acts as a folded spring to allow the heels to move apart each time the hoof is loaded and to contract each time the hoof is raised, assisting in initial shock absorption. Loading the frog actively helps push the heels apart.

The shape of the frog, both on the inside and out, is a flexible fold. This allows the width of the hoof to shorten and lengthen each time the horse takes a step, and the heels to move independently of one another. This constant flexing of the hoof as the horse moves contributes to the stimulus that develops healthy structure above. The independent movement of the heels allows the hoof to accommodate uneven ground.

The volume of the frog contributes to the strength of the back of the hoof. In a healthy hoof, fibro-cartilage under the frog melds with the lateral cartilage to form a continuous bundle of fibro-cartilage across the foot. This effectively creates a bridge that connects the frog, lateral cartilage and digital cushion together to make one strong superstructure.

BELOW LEFT Healthy heels, showing spring design.

BELOW RIGHT Contracted heels affecting spring design.

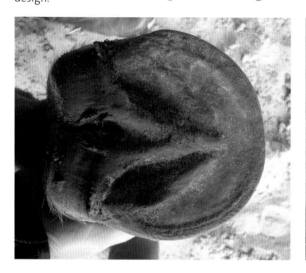
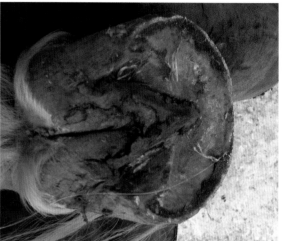

In a contracted hoof this superstructure will be severely restricted and very under-developed. In addition, the constriction caused by the narrowed area between the heels at the back of a contracted hoof can interfere with the function of veins, arteries and nerves, creating restriction of circulation, caudal heel pain and loss of sensation.

Part of the cause of this contraction seems to be the frog atrophying because of lack of stimulus. It seems as if the frog and the superstructures above it keep the heels apart when healthy. When these parts are undeveloped, the heels will tend to crush the frog and the folded spring mechanism fails, pinching the frog's central sulcus together. This area then becomes vulnerable to trapping dirt and developing infection.

Heels

A healthy hoof will always have short, strong, upright heels which appear to merge with the heel bulbs at the back of the hoof.

In an unhealthy hoof, long under-run heels always go hand-in-hand with a long toe, which increases breakover. Increased breakover creates a toe-first landing and mechanical abnormality for all the structures above the hoof. As far back as 1974, Dr James Rooney had recorded that a toe-first landing

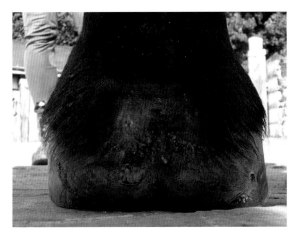 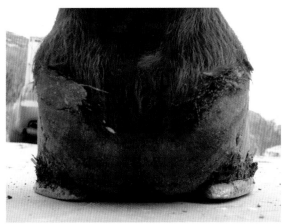

Short, upright, low heels.   The same foot 6 months previously.

impaired the way the deep flexor tendon and the fetlock joint interacted with each other.

In a heel-first landing such as one would see in a short, healthy hoof with low heels, the deep digital flexor tendon tightens as the fetlock releases tension. In a toe-first landing both the tendon and the fetlock joint tighten at the same time. The timing is subtle: get it wrong by slightly altering the point of breakover (as happens in a long toe) and you create far greater force on the navicular bone, via pressure from the deep digital flexor tendon, than Nature ever intended.

Declining hoof health

The more we look at hooves from the point of view of healthy form and structure, the more we realise that hooves which deviate from those seen on hard-working bare feet are hooves that will not function without 'protection'.

Yet this very 'protection', by shutting down the hoof's function, serves only to put the horse in a never-ending spiral of declining hoof health. Horses who land toe-first, trip, stumble, forge or are sensitive on hard surfaces, are nearer to lameness than those functioning with bare hooves over any surface at all speeds. The gradual loss of function over many years is a slow, insidious path that can lead to breakdown.

Strength of the palmar foot seems to be a vital key to good hoof health. Where this strength is compromised by under-development, improper loading of the hoof during movement and stance will result in increased stress. Peripheral loading results in under-development, so one could argue that peripheral loading causes more problems in the long term than it solves.

Future hoof potential

The role of environment, diet and exercise in contributing to the shaping of the future function and thus performance of a hoof cannot be under-estimated.

For a horse to develop the best possible hooves, he needs to receive years of stimulus on varied terrain, and to be receiving a diet that allows the feet to grow and function optimally. Dr Bowker has shown that good hooves will not reach their maximum potential or strength until the horse is about seven years old – in other words about the same time as the body reaches maturity. Early shoeing risks arresting this development and possibly weak-ening the hooves permanently.

While we continue to 'protect' our horses and their hooves from the wear and stimulus Nature designed them to respond to we cannot expect them to be truly healthy or to function optimally. We are just now seeing the potential of hooves to regain function after years of 'protection', but how much better it would be if equine professionals and horse owners were more aware of how hooves work and how they respond to stimulus, so that loss of function became a thing of the past.

5

What makes hooves change?

The starting point – unhealthy hooves

As stated at the start of this book, we turned to keeping our horses barefoot not out of inclination but because our backs were to the wall – like many people, we had lame horses whose only remaining options were retirement, a bullet or trying barefoot. These horses had been well shod over the years, but even the most conscientious farriery had been unable to prevent serious lameness.

At this stage, Fari (an eight-year-old Arab endurance horse) was off work with a suspensory ligament strain, Bailey (a five-year-old Thoroughbred cross) had severe, full depth cracks in three hooves and Ghost (a nineteen-year-old Irish Draught x Thoroughbred) had been retired owing to navicular syndrome, which had been worsening over several years despite remedial shoeing.

These horses – Fari, Bailey and Ghost – drove us to try barefoot because shoes were simply not able to keep them sound. Barefoot appeared the least of the three evils – and we decided that at least we could have the horses shod again if the experiment failed.

After much discussion, and considerable research, we removed the shoes from our horses, and set out to learn about natural hoof care. Not surprisingly, our lame horses were not rendered miraculously sound overnight. In fact, at that stage we had no real expectation that taking the shoes off would help, but it seemed worth a go, as it was one of the few things we hadn't tried.

We were also intrigued that two of our horses were totally sound without shoes. Felix (a four-year-old Irish sports horse) was, incredibly, immediately capable of hard work on all surfaces from the moment his shoes were removed. Jesta (a five-year-old Arab) had, in fact, never been shod.

That was amazing enough, but we were still no nearer to finding a way to help our other horses – in fact, at that stage we were not even sure that there was any means of improving the hooves of the three lame horses.

Problem feet; perfect feet

As we started to learn more about healthy hooves, one of the original inspirations for us (as we were both training in the US) were the hooves found on feral mustangs in Nevada and California.

These mustangs range over huge areas, and cover miles on rocky and abrasive terrain; so durable and strong are the hooves on these horses that numerous studies had been carried out by farriers, trimmers and researchers, trying to find out why they functioned so well without shoes. Their hooves were beautiful, but looked very different from the hooves on domestic horses in the UK.

One significant difference noted was that they live in desert areas – typical rainfall is very low; a totally different climate from that of Britain, where in our home area the average rainfall is 180–254 cm (70–100 in) per year.

However, like these desert mustangs, Felix and Jesta, our healthy-hooved horses at home, could cross even the most challenging surfaces at any gait or speed, in perfect comfort and without damaging their feet. This was despite our climate, and even though (unlike the mustangs) they were carrying the weight of a rider on their backs.

We believed that the key to improving the hooves on our lame horses was to find out exactly why some horses had healthier, better functioning hooves than others.

Good-looking hooves – but how do they work?

We learnt that mustang hooves had recognisable characteristics, such as a short dorsal wall length, large frogs, strong digital cushion, thick lateral cartilages and low heels.

After studying these hooves, many trimmers and farriers had set out to try to trim to this model – in other words to mimic the external appearance of a mustang hoof in their trimming, to try to create a 'mustang-type' hoof on domestic horses. They hoped that this would improve not only the appearance but also the performance of the hooves in the domestic horse.

Initially, this approach sounded like a good idea, and from a mechanical point of view it seemed a sensible strategy – if you shortened the toe, brought back an under-run heel and engaged the frog, over time it should encourage the horse's hoof to function better through improved biomechanics.

External appearance

This improvement in external appearance is typically what happens when a horse with an unhealthy foot is well shod. The farrier will try to bring the hoof print of the horse into the correct place, aiming for the horse to load his foot in the same way as he would do if the foot had grown a healthy, supportive hoof capsule.

This is beneficial in many ways. There is no doubt that a long toe and an under-run heel, together with poor foot balance, can put immense strain on the horse, as the biomechanics of the limb and hoof will be unable to function properly. Then, the harder the horse works, the greater the strain on these biomechanics. If this biomechanical strain continues beyond the age of six or seven, there is a greater risk that the horse will start to experience soft tissue injury, and may ultimately break down.

If the hoof is shod to put the hoof print of the horse in the correct place, this has a number of advantages:

- It gives better support for the limb, reducing muscle strain in the back and shoulders.

- Correct foot balance enables the horse to load his hooves evenly, reducing stress on the ligaments and tendons of the lower limb.

- A short toe allows the horse the correct breakover as he lifts his foot, improving straightness and stride length.

- Together, these factors encourage the horse to land heel first.

However, even the best shoeing also has disadvantages:

- The foot may not now be under-run, but the quality of the connection between the hoof wall and laminae has not been improved.

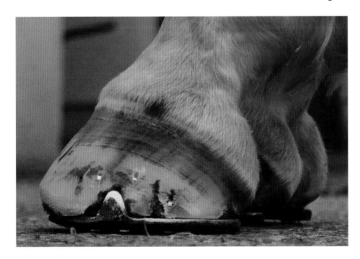

A well-shod foot. Earlier damage does not detract from the fact that the key elements of good shoeing are now in place.

- The hoof is loading peripherally, not centrally.

- The horse may land heel-first, particularly on soft ground, but the tissues in the caudal part of the hoof have not been improved and will remain under-developed.

- Stimulus to all structures is still restricted, resulting in weakness and reduced function.

- In humans, wearing shoes reduces proprioception, increases oxygen consumption, and reduces the ability of the limb to compensate for impact forces; it is likely that this is also true for horses.

Judging by appearance

The problem with good shoeing is that, although it can improve poor mechanics, it is usually addressing the symptoms of unhealthy feet (the external appearance) but not the cause.

If this is the case, then even when the mechanics have been improved, the horse may not have healthy hooves, because the internal structures of the hoof are still weak and under-stimulated. If this is the case, the horse will not be sound or comfortable on challenging surfaces, although he may cope on soft ground.

For instance, it is usually the case that a horse with high or under-run heels and long toes (see photo page 34) will have weak digital cushions and frogs. As a result, over time, the horse may start to land flat-footed, or even toe-first, because the weakness of the structures in the back of the hooves make it uncomfortable to land heel-first.

You can try this for yourself if you walk on an uncomfortable surface without shoes – you will start to land toe-first, and very quickly (unless you often wear high heels!) you will feel the strain in your calf muscles and lower back.

Landing toe-first may be more comfortable for the horse in the short term, but it loads the hoof and limb incorrectly, causing considerable strain on the tendons and ligaments of the lower limbs, particularly the deep digital flexor tendon; it can also lead to muscle tension and strain in other areas of the horse's body.

Faced with a hoof like this, most farriers and trimmers, understanding the importance of correct biomechanics, would want to shorten the toe, lower the heels, and bring the footprint of the horse back to a more supportive position under the horse. This will certainly improve both the appearance of the foot and its biomechanics, but these improvements are all external rather than internal.

In this scenario, it is likely that the horse will continue to struggle, possibly being intermittently lame, or finding uneven or rough ground uncomfortable, because the underlying essentials – the internal structures which are a prerequisite for good hoof health – are not in place.

A good trim, or a shoe, put onto a hoof like this is like a beautiful house built without foundations; it will look impressive, but will not be robust. In isolation, trimming and shoeing like this can therefore only mask the problem for a short time, if at all.

In reality, no matter how the external breakover and loading of the hoof is improved, the horse will not be comfortable to land heel-first on challenging surfaces unless, and until, the internal structures at the back of the foot (frog, digital cushion and lateral cartilages) are strengthened. In addition the horse will not grow a well-connected hoof wall unless his diet and environment are improved.

It seems, then, that even the best trimming (or shoeing) can be unproductive unless we look at the whole of the hoof, rather than just the external structures.

Common denominators of healthy hooves

We now view hooves as barometers of the overall health of the horse. Like any other part of the horse's body they can be fit or weak, healthy or sick; this status can change (sometimes very quickly) as different dietary, environmental and mechanical factors affect the hooves.

When we look at the best hooves, whether on our own horses or on feral horses, they share many physical characteristics – wide, healthy frogs, strong, smooth hoof walls, a shock-absorbing digital cushion and lateral cartilages, deep collateral grooves and good concavity.

Beyond this, though, what factors do they have in common?

Some horses with great hooves have never been shod, but equally there are unshod horses with poor feet – so this is not the answer. Some healthy-hooved horses range over many acres of dry terrain – but others are kept in wet environments such as in Wales or Ireland. Good hooves can be found on horses of different breeds, and various ages, so perhaps good hooves are just a genetic fluke?

Dynamic hooves

We used to think this might be the case, but at that stage we did not fully appreciate how dynamic a horse's hoof can be.

Over time, however, we saw again and again that horses with 'bad hooves' were trying their very hardest to grow better hooves – hooves

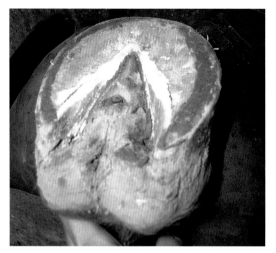 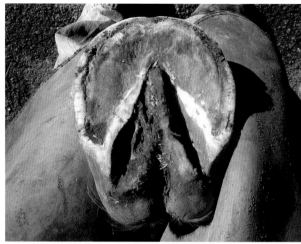

A healthy hoof can change rapidly: the right-hand photo was taken after a cycle of three shoeings caused the heels to contract.

which were biomechanically more effective, and closer to the 'healthy hooves' we saw on the best horses.

Equally, we saw that a horse's hoof could distort if the load-bearing was incorrect, and overloaded or weakened structures could result in rapid deterioration in hoof function.

> Horses have the capacity to:
>
> - Grow better-quality hoof walls.
>
> - Develop stronger digital cushions.
>
> - Strengthen their heels and frogs.
>
> - Grow thicker soles.
>
> - Improve concavity and internal hoof depth.

It is just not true that horses with bad feet are 'born' with them – but it is true that many things can conspire to damage the health of a horse's hoof, from the moment of birth.

Horses are not born lame. You don't see a 'footy' foal – foals are born with balanced, perfect feet, which are designed to be fully functional within minutes of the birth. In fact, the hoof starts to respond to stimulus almost at once.

The foal in the photo opposite shows a clear demarcation in his hoof: the hoof quality changed the day he was born as a result of the boost in circulation when he first started to move on his feet. His hooves have responded

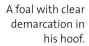
A foal with clear demarcation in his hoof.

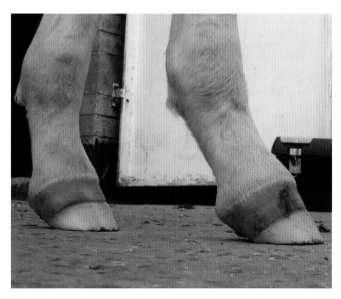

to the improved circulation with stronger growth – a clear illustration of how essential movement is for healthy hooves.

There is another crucial advantage which foals have over many adult domestic horses: a foal is supplied a completely balanced diet, via the dam's milk. This ensures that the foal has all the vitamins, minerals and essential nutrients required in order to grow and support healthy feet.

Despite this good starting-point, as we have seen in the previous chapter, many horses' hooves deteriorate over the years (or in some cases never fully develop), even to the point where the horse becomes lame as a result.

Understanding that hooves are dynamic, we now see that if they can improve, they can also deteriorate. Genetics are the one constant during a horse's life, so it is unarguable that, for many horses, their bad hooves are made, not born.

The next question, of course, is to find out what is actually happening to poor hooves to make them fail. If we know what causes this, we can try to reverse the process.

Creating unhealthy hooves

An ironic fact is that the more expensive a horse is, the more we will tend to cosset and confine him. As a result, the hooves on some of the most highly priced horses receive little or no challenge or stimulus, from birth onwards. These hooves are likely to be under-developed and weak in the adult horse.

By contrast, a feral Exmoor foal, worth only a few pounds, will roam on challenging surfaces from his day of birth and, if this carries on throughout life, he will develop much healthier hooves, giving him a better prognosis for long-term soundness.

Assessing our own and our clients' horses, it became clear that our lame horses had received the wrong kind of management for developing optimum hooves.

Thus we learnt that the recipe for *unhealthy* hooves is as follows:

- Restrict movement, particularly from a young age, while the hoof is growing and developing, so the horse's hooves have no need to become fit or strong.

- Allow the horse to live and work on only the softest, least challenging surfaces so that the digital cushion and frog will atrophy and the fibro-cartilage necessary for optimum health will fail to develop. Grassy fields, rubber matting or deep stable beds are the best 'soft option' for horses' hooves.

- Ensure that the horse has a diet which supplies more sugar and protein than he requires. Ad lib grazing on green, UK pasture, particularly in spring and summer, is almost guaranteed to achieve this.

- Make sure the diet lacks minerals, further compromising the horse's metabolism and, ultimately, hoof integrity. Many UK pastures are deficient in key minerals so grazing twenty-four hours a day without supplementation will be an extremely unhealthy option for most hooves.

- Keep hooves wet. Constant wet weather allows hooves to be under almost constant attack from bacteria and fungi. Although a healthy hoof can deal well with periodic wet weather and work on wet ground, a hoof that rarely has the chance to be on dry, well-drained ground will be a hoof thoroughly under stress. The UK climate in many areas is both wet and humid, so hooves here will rarely lack moisture and are often stressed in this way.

- Shoe the horse before the internal structures of the hoof are fully developed. Research shows that horses' hooves take as long as the rest of their bodies to develop fully – and most horses are not fully mature until seven or eight years of age. Shoeing before a horse is seven or eight years old plays an important role in arresting the development of the digital cushions and frogs. Shoeing onto an already healthy hoof for short periods is not as effective in causing damage, as a healthy hoof will retain much of its proper function.

- Shoe or trim the horse in a way that interferes with natural hoof function or with medial/lateral balance so that risk of soft tissue injuries, particularly tendon or ligament strain, is increased. Raising the frog off the ground and ensuring that the horse has long toes or high heels is the best way to cause a horse to land toe-first, encourage tripping, and create inflammation of the deep digital flexor tendon and navicular bursa.

- Load the hoof peripherally so that, over time, the pedal bone will lose density and integrity. Constantly loading the hoof on its periphery is very successful in causing biomechanical problems and eventual lameness later on in the horse's life.

Our own horses taught us that it was probable that horses could accommodate or adapt to poor biomechanics to a certain extent, and that most would remain injury free while they were still young. However, over the longer term, and on tougher surfaces, the adaptations required by poor biomechanics obviously caused undue strain on other structures of the hoof and limb and could lead to eventual lameness.

We have noticed that there seems to be a pattern amongst many of the horses who come to us lame from hoof or related limb problems (for example caudal pain, 'navicular', tendonitis or ligament strains). These horses are typically between eight to ten years old, and have usually had intermittent or recurrent lameness for a period of several months, or even longer.

For example, out of the horses with hoof-related lameness whom we have rehabilitated in the two years prior to writing this book, 80 per cent were between six and ten years of age and 90 per cent had been intermittently lame for at least six months – though some had been lame for much longer.

All these horses returned to full soundness barefoot within three to six months of rehabilitation.

Hooves where the worst has happened

As horse owners we were aware of the problems that affected horses' hooves – the most well-known historically being navicular syndrome and laminitis.

However, poor hoof development and impaired biomechanics are also commonly responsible for tendon, ligament and bone damage.

The suspensory and sesamoidean ligaments, the deep digital flexor tendon and the navicular and pedal bones are particularly vulnerable.

Textbooks tend to view these problems in isolation, but in reality they share a common basis, where whole hoof health and therefore whole hoof function has been compromised and has ultimately broken down.

'Navicular syndrome'/caudal pain/deep digital flexor tendonitis

Although 'navicular syndrome' is a widely used term, recent studies[10] have shown that horses presenting with the pattern of lameness typical of 'navicular syndrome' only occasionally have damage to the navicular bone itself.

In fact, on MRI (magnetic resonance imaging) these horses are more frequently seen to be suffering from soft tissue injuries, particularly to the deep digital flexor tendon, rather than from bone damage.

The more traditional route to a 'navicular' diagnosis is the path followed by Copper, a Trakehner competing at Medium level dressage (and by countless other horses in the UK before and since).

Copper's lameness manifested itself very gradually, and he would go through periods of apparent soundness, followed by intermittent lameness, with shortened strides. Initially his lameness was most evident on hard ground and on tight circles, but as his condition deteriorated, the lameness became chronic.

The diagnosis was made on the basis of nerve blocks to the caudal third of the foot (as a result of which he came sound) and radiographs which showed changes to the navicular bone.

Historically, as with Copper, radiographs were the usual precursor to a 'navicular' diagnosis as, in horse with this type of lameness, they often showed areas of degeneration in the navicular bone.

This was not a totally reliable diagnostic though, as many mature horses had some bone degeneration without apparent lameness, and lame horses could have navicular bones that looked fine on radiograph.

The most recent studies confirm earlier research[11] which proposed that damage to the navicular bone is the last stage of the degenerative process, only occurring after the deep digital flexor tendon and navicular bursa have become damaged and inflamed as a consequence of poor biomechanics and under-development of the fibro-cartilage in the back of the hoof.

Today, when MRI can be used, it shows up these areas of inflammation clearly, even when bony changes are not apparent on radiographs. As a result, horses with the pattern of lameness shown by Copper will, on examination by MRI, often be shown to have lesions or inflammation of the deep digital flexor tendon. In the most severe cases, damage may be also evident in the navicular bone, but this is now believed to be a consequence of prolonged soft tissue damage rather than a distinct condition.

As a result, radiographs showing changes in the navicular bone alone are now viewed as an inconsistent basis for diagnosis, but MRI is expensive and is unavailable for many horses.

For several years, Copper's owner kept the lameness more or less at bay with remedial shoeing and drug therapy, but he gradually got worse until he seemed headed for an early retirement.

When his shoes came off, he had a weak back of the foot, with a poor digital cushion and weak lateral cartilages. Contracted and under-run heels further compromised the back of his hoof. These factors, together with his long toes, had given him a toe-first landing which may have led to his problems, since a toe-first landing puts the deep digital flexor tendon under inappropriate strain.

His owner was concerned that going barefoot would not work for him, as he had always been very sore when he lost a shoe, but, like so many others, she felt she had few alternatives.

The key to returning Copper to soundness was to improve the health of the back of his foot.

Once his shoes were off, this involved him working on surfaces which he found comfortable, so that his frog could start to engage without being subjected to undue pressure.

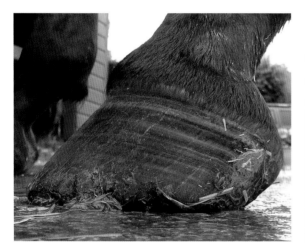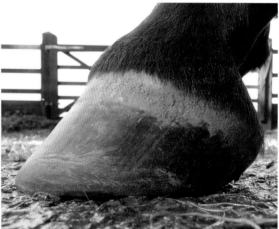

Over time this allowed his heels, along with his frog, to broaden and decontract. The combination of frog pressure and proper stimulation from supportive surfaces started to rebuild his digital cushion and lateral cartilages. As these began to strengthen, it became possible for Copper to start to engage the back of his foot again, breaking the cycle that had first made him lame.

ABOVE LEFT Copper with under-run heels.

ABOVE RIGHT Copper's same hoof one year later.

Once the back of his foot was healthier, he started to land heel-first, which relieved the stress on his deep digital flexor tendon and, in turn, on the navicular bursa.

At the same time, his diet and environment had been improved. This was essential, as the dietary changes relieved his sole sensitivity and allowed for a better-connected hoof capsule to grow in, at a steeper angle. This shortened his long toe, which had inevitably accompanied his long heels, improving his breakover and the biomechanics of both his hoof and lower limb.

A more challenging and stimulating environment provided physiotherapy for his hooves, while keeping him comfortable.

It took six months of this regime to return Copper to soundness, but once he was able to work consistently he made rapid progress.

Our experience is that if problems are picked up early, when the horse initially becomes lame, then often only soft tissue damage is involved and it can be reversed fairly quickly.

In another case, a six-year-old horse described as short-striding and bilaterally lame, arrived for rehabilitation. He was clearly landing toe-first, but this was a relatively recent problem. Within two weeks of starting rehabilitation he was landing heel-first and was level, with a good stride length, on all but the most challenging surfaces. It took only a very short time for him to begin to use himself correctly because the damage had been caught at an early stage.

By contrast, a twelve-year-old horse, who had been lame for nearly eighteen months, took much longer – four months – before he was no longer lame on supportive ground. In his case, soft tissue damage over a prolonged period had led to significant bone damage as well. In addition, he had been shod for so many years that the structures of the back of his foot were very weak, and took much longer to rehabilitate.

The effects of laminitis

As mentioned in Chapter 3, collateral groove depth is a good indicator of hoof health in most hooves, but care is needed in assessing laminitic hooves, which can have deep collateral grooves despite being weak and damaged.

In these hooves, what appears to be collateral groove depth occurs where the pedal bone has 'rotated', giving an illusion of depth at the back of the hoof. The giveaway is that, unlike in a healthy hoof, the rest of the sole may have no or little concavity. In addition, the hoof will always have a stretched white line, with ripples and distortion in the hoof wall and a sharp angled deviation when the dorsal wall is viewed from the side.

In a laminitic hoof, the hoof wall connection is weak. The attachment of the hoof wall to the internal structures is lost, and the hoof wall starts to detach (shown by a stretched white line and dorsal wall deviation – see photo in the section Wall Deviation, page 28). In the most serious cases of laminitis, the pedal bone can even penetrate the sole. If, as seems to be the case, the sole is well able to support part of the weight of the horse when it is healthy, then there must be a catastrophic lack of integrity in the attachment of the sole (just as in the dorsal wall) to allow the pedal bone to penetrate in this way.

Typically, one of the first precursors of laminitis (which literally means 'inflammation of the laminae') is sole sensitivity, which is more readily evident in a barefoot horse than a shod horse. We believe from our own observations that the sole is as much compromised as the hoof wall during an attack of laminitis.

Without the support of a well-connected hoof wall, mechanical force and the weight of the horse puts undue pressure on the sole, resulting in the sole stretching, thinning and flattening. The thickness and depth which, in a healthy sole, protect the solar corium are lost and the horse will begin to find the pinpoint pressure of uneven ground uncomfortable.

White soles occasionally have black areas, which can be areas of pigment. However, on dissection and microscopic examination, Mark Johnson (a dual qualified farrier and UK Natural Hoof Care Practitioner) has found that some black patches are areas of necrotic tissue. These are always found in hooves with poor laminar connection, and he theorises that the necrosis may be the result of compression and solar corium damage which has been caused by incorrect suspension of the internal structures. These black areas can reduce or even disappear as hooves become healthier.

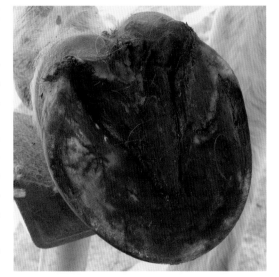

Black necrosis: black patches are areas of necrotic tissue.

Other metabolic issues

Insulin resistance has recently started to be recognised as a cause of metabolic problems in the horse, and these types of horses are some of the most challenging horses to take barefoot.

The hoof is always a barometer of the overall health of the horse, and so a compromised metabolism will always mean a compromised hoof. One of the advantages of having such horses barefoot, however, is that the owner has very clear feedback about the horse's health status, and what is affecting it.

Sam is a horse with metabolic issues, and as is commonly the case, his owner had no idea that anything was wrong until his shoes came off. He had weak, flat feet, with poorly developed digital cushions, like many horses who have been shod for prolonged periods, but there seemed no reason why they should not improve, as his owner was an experienced barefooter who already had other horses who were doing well out of shoes.

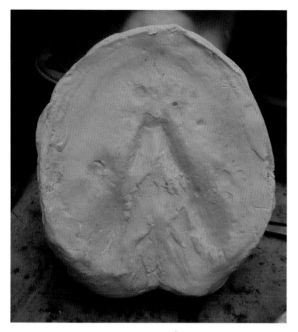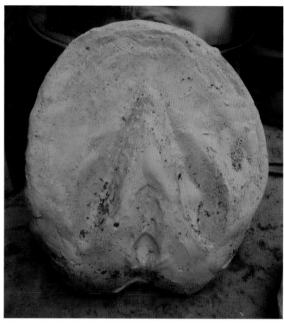

Plaster casts of Sam's hooves in May (ABOVE LEFT) and November (ABOVE RIGHT).

Sam was fed a good diet, which perfectly suited his owner's other horses, and which should have met all his nutritional needs. His feet were not capable of work without boots initially, but over a period of months, his hooves developed and improved, and he was working happily barefoot. Plaster casts of his hoof (see photos) show its progress over a period of five months.

In the autumn he was wormed (there were no other changes in his diet or routine), and forty-eight hours later he suffered severe sole sensitivity and was trying to relieve his discomfort by walking on the back halves of his feet. Again, plaster casts were taken and these demonstrated quite clearly that not just his sole but the whole integrity of his hoof capsule had been compromised.

The plaster casts track the effects: the initial sole sensitivity is followed by damage to the laminae, which allows the internal structures of the hoof to collapse. Externally, the hoof goes from being short and concave, with deep collateral grooves, a strong frog and well-developed heel and back of the foot, to being flatter, with a weak frog, shallow collateral grooves and stretched toe.

Wormers were not the only things to trigger this sensitivity. Over the next year he suffered similar setbacks after exposure to commercially farmed ryegrass and, later in the same year, even to too much meadow grass. With horses like this, there can seem to be a cumulative build-up, so that they become more sensitive after several attacks, rather like an allergic reaction.

These horses can grow healthy hooves successfully, but their owners and trimmers need to be extremely careful about monitoring the diet and the chemicals they are exposed to.

Sole sensitivity

Eric is a former grade-A show-jumper and hunter, whose owners, like many of us, took his shoes off as a last resort.

Eric had been intermittently lame for some time, and had been turned away as there was no clear cause for his lameness. His farrier was understandably worried about him coming out of shoes, because his soles were so sensitive that he could not even stand happily unshod. When he was shod, the only way to keep him comfortable was for the front shoes to be immediately replaced before his hind shoes were removed.

As with most horses, the first thing to be addressed was his diet. UK Natural Hoof Care Practitioners routinely discuss each new horse's diet in detail eight weeks or more before shoes come off. We find that this minimises sole sensitivity in horses coming out of shoes, and in most cases allows horses to go straight from shoes to working barefoot.

Eric had ripples in his hoof wall and shallow collateral grooves, a sure sign that his hoof wall connection was compromised. This is usually a result of mineral deficiencies or a diet too rich in non-structural carbohydrates. As this normally gives rise to sole sensitivity as well (as in Eric's case), it was essential to change his diet before taking his shoes off.

Out of shoes, and after a few weeks on a revised diet, he was immediately able to stand without shoes, which was already an improvement on his previous comfort level. In fact he was so much more comfortable that he could work straight away on soft surfaces or smooth, hard surfaces.

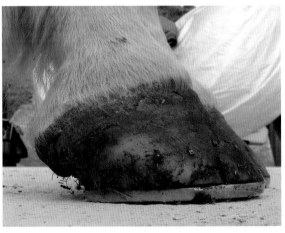

Eric in shoes.

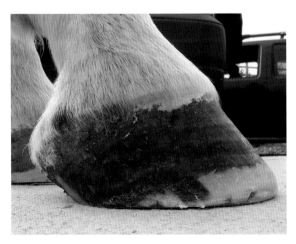

Eric 4 months later.

However, as the back of his foot was weak, with a poor digital cushion and under-run heels, his owner was warned that it would take time before he was capable of working without protection on hard, stony ground.

Over the next three to four months, his hooves strengthened to the point that he could cope with even stony ground, and as with all horses, consistent work was a key factor in building his new, stronger hooves.

His owner is also now extremely careful with his diet, and views any deterioration in the performance of his hooves as a sure sign that he is getting too much rich grass.

By restricting his grazing as necessary, perhaps allowing him access to grazing only at night, she can put a stop to his sole sensitivity, and the damage to his hoof capsule that would inevitably result.

Ligament and tendon damage

We have already seen how poor hoof function can affect the deep digital flexor tendon and the ligaments within the hoof; equally the rest of the horse's body will be directly affected by the health, or otherwise, of his hooves.

A healthy hoof protects the soft tissue of the limb above by effectively absorbing shock and dissipating the tremendous energy produced by the horse's limbs landing at speed.

If the hoof is unhealthy, however, and unable to perform this function, energy has to be absorbed elsewhere, putting extra strain on the ligaments and tendons of the distal limb, which already function close to maximum load when the horse is galloping.

If the horse is also shod, lack of proprioception means that the hoof is not as capable of adapting to impact forces or compensating for uneven ground.

It's not surprising, therefore, that horses with unhealthy feet, and particularly those in shoes, are at greater risk of soft tissue injury.

Charlie is a horse who had suffered from being shod as a four-year-old. Lack of proprioception, poor shock absorption and a heel imbalance in his hooves had put severe strain on him. Although he was only in very light work, he went lame first in his right fore then left fore from strain to his check ligaments.

As with the other horses in the previous examples, however, his problem was not simply mechanics, but was exacerbated by a poor diet, which had prevented him from growing the best possible hoof.

His hoof wall was poorly attached, which will have exaggerated the biomechanical problems caused by the shoes, since a weak hoof wall is less able to resist incorrect loading forces.

Although his hooves appeared externally to be fine, when his diet was improved there was a clear demarcation in his hooves, and the dorsal hoof wall could clearly be seen growing in at a much steeper angle. As with Eric, the sole sensitivity he had initially showed disappeared, and he also became much calmer.

Charlie's workload was increased once he was totally sound. Since then, he has covered many miles on challenging, steep and uneven terrain, and his check ligaments have not subsequently caused him any problems.

Charlie is a classical case of a horse whose hooves are perfectly adapted to suit him; his hooves work extremely effectively but did not do so when human ideas of loading and balance were imposed on him.

Hoof problems: holistic, not simplistic

The common theme here is that hoof problems are not normally caused by a single disease or failure. Hoof function is founded on a good diet, which allows a hoof to grow and maintain its integrity, and an environment that stimulates and strengthens the whole hoof. Healthy hooves and correct biomechanical function are intrinsically linked to each other and interdependent.

6

What can healthy hooves achieve?

> Domestication ensured that horses as we would come to think of them would not be horses in their natural setting, nor behaving in their natural fashion. Humans would inevitably see horses through their dreams and ambitions, myths and fears, vanities and fashions.
>
> Stephen Budiansky, *The Nature of Horses*, 1997

Even though our horses may benefit from being kept as naturally as possible, most of us want to do all sorts of 'unnatural' things with them – not least riding and competing. Barefoot has to be more than a natural option – it has to be a performance option.

Throughout the world, we can find horses with fantastic, healthy hooves. We believe that, generally, horses have healthy hooves the minute that they are born – whether they stay that way then depends on how they live. With horses who have healthy hooves throughout their lives, there are factors which they all have in common.

These healthy hooved horses:

- Are on a diet which is suitable for their evolution and biology.

- Cover many miles on their bare hooves over a variety of terrain.

- Self-maintain their hoof balance with minor human intervention.

The first two criteria obviously apply perfectly to feral or wild horses, but they, and the third, are equally true of the best-performing barefoot domesticated horses. Whether a feral horse or a riding horse, the horse's basic biology and physiology remain the same; therefore the criteria for hoof health is similar whether your horse is a Warmblood or mustang. Because of the differences in conformation and appearance between different breeds of horse, this can sometimes be hard for us to accept.

We've therefore included this chapter as an inspiration to anyone who might be considering taking their horse out of shoes, but who is worrying about whether horses can really perform barefoot.

We, our fellow hoof care practitioners and our clients have horses who work and compete in every discipline. The feedback from riders is consistent – they believe their horses actually perform *better* than when they were shod.

As barefoot horses currently form only a minority of the working horse population, by comparison with shod horses, there are relatively few such horses competing at affiliated levels at present. However, those who do are performing extremely well.

Perhaps more importantly, riders who have now spent some years competing on barefoot horses (at the same level as they previously competed on shod horses) are finding that their horses are maintaining their soundness for longer. Injury and breakdown rates are extremely low, not only on a daily basis, but consistently from season to season.

Barefoot eventing

The fantastic ability of bare hooves to absorb shock, and their enhanced proprioception, means that they are perfect for going cross-country, whether the going is deep or hard.

It is very common for riders to worry about not having studs the first time they go cross-country on a barefoot horse. The horses, however, have no such concerns.

> Dear old Tetley has just flown round our nearest course, Henbury Hall, clear all the way. It was a very big course, but technically not difficult so I just went for it and jumped pretty much everything without slowing down at all. He made it seem very small! ... I heard a rider with two studs in each shoe say, 'It's *very* slippery out there', to another rider. There had been a steady drizzle all morning and people were very afraid of the going. We didn't slip once!'
>
> Caroline Trayes, competing at Novice level in 2005

> Appallingly slippy going…watched the person before me skid two whole strides into a fence and wipe out…not good for one's confidence when those with studs do that…
>
> Jane Tweedie, competing at a Pre-novice event in 2007 (she went clear, won the class and she and her barefoot horse came home five seconds under the time!)

Jane Tweedie eventing successfully barefoot.

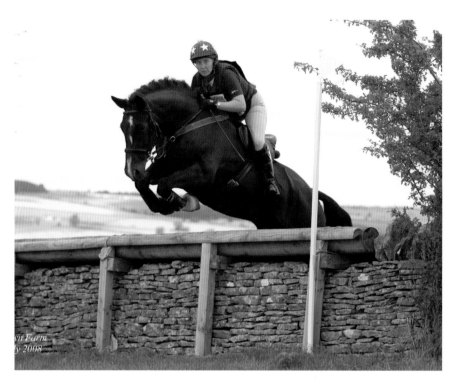

Barefoot endurance

Endurance is a discipline where barefoot horses succeeded from the early days and perhaps confounded the critics the most. Worldwide, barefoot horses have covered thousands and thousands of competitive miles, over all conceivable types of terrain.

Here in the UK, Les Sparks was the first person to achieve 100 miles barefoot with his horse Jasper. Co-author Sarah was inspired by this achievement to keep her own horse, Jesta, working without shoes, and this started her on her barefoot journey. Another successful rider was Terry Madden:

> Abu baffled everyone. He had recurrent lameness problems, which had been investigated using nerve blocks, MRI and gamma scans, but the vets were unable to diagnose a specific cause. In the November he came out of shoes and then competed in the following March. The photograph [page 77] shows him at this competitive ride, which he completed with a grade 1 over a distance of 40 km [25 miles]. Since then, among other successes, he has been placed second in a 120 km [75 mile] race ride at speeds of 15 km [9⅓ miles] per hour.
>
> Spurred on by Abu's success, and the lessons learned, all our horses have now been barefoot for the last four years. Being barefoot has not stopped me competing at Advanced level. Indeed, Abu is still competing whilst his rivals seem to have disappeared, retired usually due to lameness.

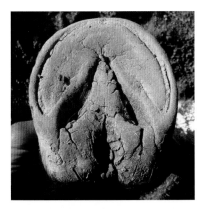

One of Halkim's front hooves after 105 miles of barefoot riding in Southern Utah in one weekend, no boots! No kidding!'

[Comment by Kirt Lander of the USA, who kindly supplied this photo.]

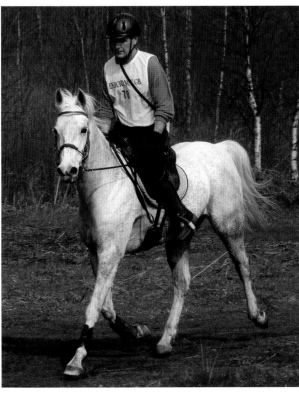

Abu had a history of undiagnosed lameness but, since coming out of shoes, he has been competing successfully in endurance rides, and remains sound.

Mehdraar is my youngster who competed in a 50 km [30 mile] ride at Lindum. He won Best Novice Horse within the Cheshire and North Wales Endurance Group in his first season.

> Terry Madden, who competes his barefoot endurance horses in the UK.

Helen Newton had the following to say about her horses:

Carly first broke down in 2001 at the age of seven with check ligament and tendon strains in both forelegs. After long periods of box rest and slowly bringing him back into work several times, only for him to become lame again, it was suggested by the vets that his problems could be due to hoof imbalance. My farrier was only interested in shoeing, so I called in a specialist hoof trimmer. It turned out that Carly had sheared, contracted heels that were too high, plus severe medial/lateral imbalance. Five years on, after bringing him gradually back into the work he loves – endurance – he won the 28-mile free speed Sport Endurance ride held at Formby, Lancashire. Although the picture shown is taken on a long stretch of sandy beach, the ride covered varied terrain including smooth tarmac, stony tracks, grassy paths, soft sand dunes as well as the firm sand of the beach, all this completely barefoot. Carly hacks regularly, competes in endurance rides up to 30 miles and can turn his hoof to a decent dressage test. We occasionally use hoof boots on his fronts if the going is likely to include a lot of hard and stony tracks.

My other horse had his shoes removed the day he arrived, aged five, having probably worn them for at least a year. He had 'bull-nosed' hinds, low heels, weak digital cushions and fairly flat soles. I used hoof boots on him all that summer and still use them when necessary. His hooves are improving all the time, with thick, concave soles and a strong digital cushion. He has been successful at low-level endurance up to 30 miles, the high point so far being winning the Sport Endurance 20-mile free speed 'Jacques' ride in Staffordshire in July 2007. Unfortunately we lost time retracing our steps to retrieve a missing boot in the 2008 ride and completed the last 5 miles of the ride completely barefoot, still achieving fourth place! This could have been a different story had it been a nailed-on metal shoe that we had lost. He is hacked out regularly, has flatwork sessions in the firmest of sand arenas and enjoys fast cross-country rides and jumping – all barefoot.

Helen Newton, endurance rider

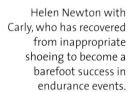

Helen Newton with Carly, who has recovered from inappropriate shoeing to become a barefoot success in endurance events.

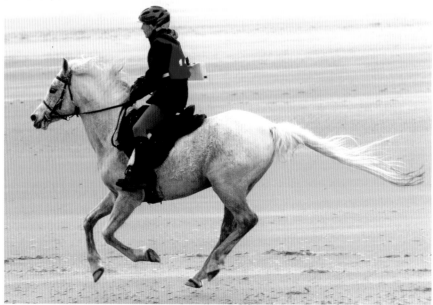

The Australian endurance rider, Jenny Moncur, observed:

> A lot of people have been sitting back and watching what happens with barefoot, but with many of the above riders placing or winning, as well as winning best conditioned awards, it is obvious that not only can it be done, but it can be done competitively too.
>
> The other interesting thing I have noticed with this current mare and my previous endurance horse is that their heart rates are consistently lower. Both of my mares have logbooks from their shod endurance days, and I also have results from their barefoot days. In both cases, heart rates are lower both pre-ride and at vet-checks. It is very noticeable by a factor of up to ten beats post-ride. Other barefooters I have spoken to have commented on the same thing.
>
> Jenny Moncur, Australian endurance rider

Barefoot Hunting

Hunting is one of the most challenging sports for any horse. It takes place during the autumn and winter months, when the ground is often wet and deep; and the nature of hunting is that you never know quite what terrain you will travel over, how far you will go or what jumps you will encounter. You and you horse might end up going along several miles of roads, or along stony tracks; you might spend hours on ploughed fields or wet moorland; you might cross rivers or jump hedges.

Typically, on a day's hunting, at least one of the shod horses in the field will lose shoes as a consequence of the ground conditions, which usually means an early end to the day.

Hunting was actually one of the first sports that Nic tried without shoes, and she hunts on Exmoor. There is little jumping on Exmoor, but lots of challenging terrain, with sharp, flinty tracks, and unforgiving stony ground.

A frequent question from riders of shod horses is: how do we manage to negotiate this type of terrain without shoes? It is assumed that our unshod horses will damage their feet on the flints.

In fact, of course, on ground like this a shoe offers little protection; the hoof wall is reinforced by a metal band, but (with standard shoeing) most of the horse's sole and frog are exposed. Whether shod or barefoot, horses need to have robust, healthy soles to cover such ground in comfort, and horses who lack this will often suffer bruising.

However, over hundreds of days on the moor, and thousands of miles, Nic's horses' feet have been unharmed, and in fact she believes they have simply become stronger and healthier with work on these challenging surfaces.

Barefoot hunting.

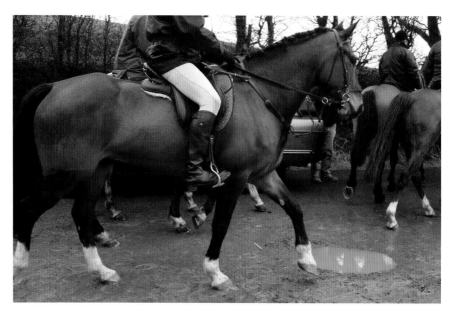

Competing successfully in cross-country driving, barefoot.

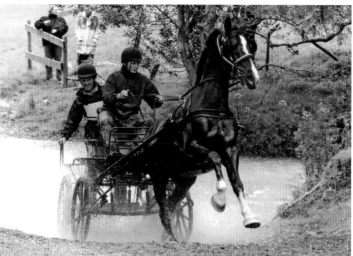

Other disciplines barefoot

Many of our dressage riders whose horses go barefoot report better balance and movement from their horses. Going barefoot can also work well for driving horses, as the photo above shows.

Experiments with barefoot racing

One racing yard tried an experiment in racing horses barefoot, focusing primarily on the trim. As they were unable or unwilling to change the diet and environment of their horses, they found that they needed to return to using metal shoes in order to improve their horses' comfort levels and performance.

Interestingly, one of the reasons they used as an argument for returning to shoes was that one of their horses seemed to be reluctant to jump owing, it was presumed, to the fear of slipping. The belief was that once this horse had metal shoes on his feet, he would then have much better traction and go back to jumping with confidence. He was therefore shod, but during his next race this horse was pulled up and, although he has raced since, his results have been disappointing.

We have not seen the horse, and so we can only theorise about what might actually have happened. However, our experience is that horses who are fed a high-cereal, high-sugar, high-starch diet (as many racehorses are) will frequently suffer from foot discomfort and sole sensitivity. Over the medium term, such a diet can lead to the hoof capsule itself becoming distorted and weakened, losing concavity and therefore traction. By this stage, the hoof's function and the horse's performance are both likely to be compromised, and simply putting a metal shoe onto such a hoof was obviously not sufficient to solve the problem.

7

Diet and feeding for the healthiest hooves

Diet has a profound effect on the hooves of horses. It would be impossible to write a book about barefoot performance without including dietary dos and don'ts, because if your horse's diet is wrong, your horse's hoof health will be seriously compromised.

As diet is so important, all UKNHCP practitioners and students receive specific training on all aspects of equine nutrition and how it can affect the hoof. We advise our clients about their horses' diets as a fundamental part of our hoof care practices, and the advice and support of independent nutritionists is vital.

All the dietary advice in this chapter is tried and tested on our own performance horses, and has been checked by an independent nutritionist, but every horse is different. Your horse's health and soundness are *always* the best guides to whether a particular diet is right for him, and you should seek advice from your vet and from a nutritionist if you have any concerns about your horse's diet.

A natural, balanced diet

As horse owners, we acknowledge the truism that a complete and balanced diet is essential for our horses, but often without fully appreciating the dramatic effects of diet specifically on hooves.

The good news is that dietary improvement can affect hooves just as quickly as dietary disasters, and that common problems are easy to correct.

Sensitive systems

Some horses are particularly sensitive to dietary imbalance, and within any group of horses on the same diet and management regime, there will be

> **A few facts you may not know about diet and hooves:**
>
> - A diet high in non-structural carbohydrates can turn a sound horse into a 'footy' horse in a matter of hours.
>
> - Mineral deficiencies can give a horse with beautiful-looking hooves painful sole sensitivity.
>
> - In a barefoot horse, you get earlier feedback about dietary problems than in a shod horse. Sole sensitivity is often the earliest warning sign and is picked up sooner in a horse whose feet are not peripherally loaded.

some who react much more quickly to problems than others – we call these the 'canaries in the coal-mine', as they often provide an early warning that all is not well.

Equally, there will be other horses, like Jesta and Felix, who remain sound and happy on challenging surfaces despite a less-than-perfect diet.

It's rather like us – we have all heard of people who live to a ripe old age despite eating lots of fatty foods and rarely eating enough fruit and vegetables, but across the population as a whole, those who eat healthily will generally have fewer long-term health problems.

In reality, as with people, it's about feeding your horse a biologically appropriate diet.

Natural environment and diet

Horses (and of course their hooves) evolved to function on a fibrous, low-sugar diet, which could only be found by roaming over large areas. Given the choice, horses prefer a variety of forage including grasses, sedges and shrubs which includes large amounts of insoluble fibre, with a low percentage of non-structural carbohydrates. Non-structural carbohydrates should not constitute a large part of a horse's diet. Examples of non-structural carbohydrates include fructans (which are nutritionally classed in this way despite being technically fibre), starch and sugars.

Searching for food and movement are therefore closely linked, with feral horses moving considerable distances each day to find food, and spending around 70 per cent of their time grazing and foraging.

Horses survive extremely well on diets based on high-fibre forage, which is low in soluble carbohydrate. They have evolved to thrive in areas where ruminants, such as cattle and sheep, would struggle to survive.[12] Ruminants digest food very efficiently, but it takes them much longer than horses to complete the digestive process. There is a limit to how much food a ruminant can digest over a given time and, on poor quality forage, their digestive system slows down even more.

By contrast, a horse will do very well on a higher fibre, lower feed value diet since, even though he cannot digest it as efficiently as a ruminant, he can digest a greater quantity of food in order to obtain enough energy.

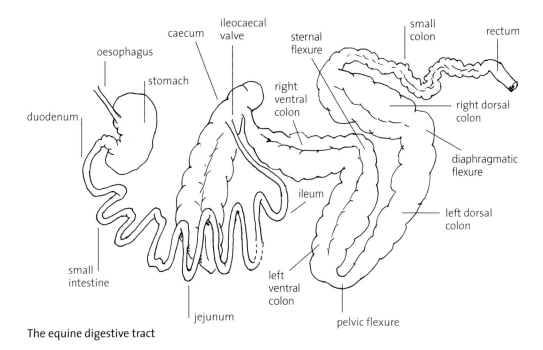

The equine digestive tract

The domesticated diet

In domestication, however, we tend not to respect this fundamental difference between horses and cattle or sheep, nor to remember that the horse evolved to continuously consume large amounts of stemmy plants which are low in nutrients.

Instead, we feed horses on farmed grasses, whether as pasture or as hay. This type of forage tends to be higher in fructans (and other non-structural carbohydrates) and protein than the horse would eat naturally. Lower in fibre, these grasses have often been selected to be suitable for increasing milk yield or weight gain in ruminants. For example, ryegrass, which ironically is often farmed for horses, is particularly high in fructans.

In addition, farmed pastures contain a more restricted range of plants than would occur naturally. In this environment, therefore, a horse will have access to less biodiversity than in the habitat in which he evolved to live.

Problems of starch overload

As if this is not enough, we frequently bring in another challenge to our horses' digestive systems. We supplement their diets with compound feeds, containing sugars and cereals (oats, barley, maize, etc.), which are low in fibre, high in starch and difficult for horses to digest when fed in large quantities. The harder our horses are working, the greater the proportion of compound feeds we feel they need.

The problem here is that, although horses can digest starch, they can only do so safely in limited quantities. Starch-digesting enzymes are found only in the small intestine, so if horses are overfed starch, some will pass into the hindgut without being properly digested.[13] Here, bacteria which feed on starch increase rapidly and cause it to ferment, and this can lead to the hindgut becoming acidic. This excess acidity can cause metabolic and hoof problems, including colic and laminitis, and the disruption to the hindgut can also cause the release of toxins into the blood and problems with absorption of nutrients.

So, in domestication, we typically reverse the ratio between soluble and insoluble carbohydrate, giving the horse large amounts of non-structural carbohydrates but insufficient overall dietary fibre.

For example, short-cropped UK spring grass can contain up to 25 per cent non-structural carbohydrates in the form of fructans, but has low levels of fibre. Horses kept solely on this type of pasture are already at risk of dietary and hoof problems, and this risk increases if they are also fed

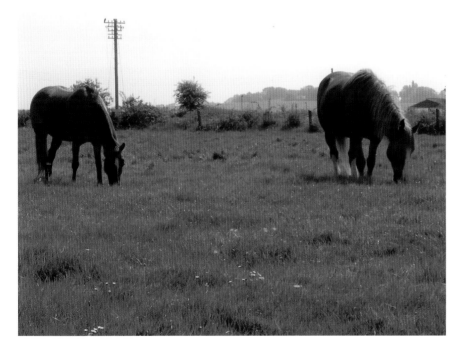

Typical spring pasture in the UK.

additional non-structural carbohydrate in the form of the starches or sugars found in hard feed.

The further we stray from the horse's natural diet, the greater the strain we put on our horses' systems. One of the first places that problems show up is in the horse's hooves.

Admittedly, understanding of equine nutritional needs has improved radically over the last few years. Most of us are now aware that horses do best on ad lib forage, both from a physiological and behavioural point of view. Most of us are also aware that a horse must have sufficient minerals in his diet in order to grow healthy hooves.

In practice, though, what does this really mean?

Diet for the barefoot horse

For barefoot horses and their owners diet quickly becomes the most fundamental element in hoof health, and for those of us with barefoot performance horses it would be no exaggeration to say that diet is almost an obsession!

Why? Because diet can make or break a hoof, and can turn a healthy hoof into an unhealthy one in a matter of hours.

It takes a little longer to restore health to a hoof that has suffered diet-related damage: days (or sometimes weeks) rather than hours, but the improvements can be equally remarkable. This may sound melodramatic, but it's something that we see time and time again in almost every horse we encounter – whether barefoot or shod.

Sarah's young horse, Morris, was sent to a professional trainer to be backed over a four-week period in early summer. During this time, the trainer planned to keep Morris and six other young horses on a 7-acre mixed pasture of leafy, 15–20 cm (6–8 in) grasses. At home, Morris had a diet low in non-structural carbohydrates with ad lib forage but limited access to grass, and he had always been very sound on challenging surfaces.

Ten days into Morris' training, turned out in this pasture 24/7, the trainer reported that Morris had initially become footsore and after a few more days was lame. At this point, three of the other young horses were also 'footy' and the trainer's solution was to have them shod in front.

Since Sarah preferred not to shoe Morris, she asked the trainer to restrict his grazing and provide ad lib hay instead. Within a few days, Morris was no longer lame but was still not totally comfortable on challenging surfaces. Two weeks later, though, he had recovered full hoof health.

Frequently, inadequate diets are also lacking in the right levels of key minerals, or the minerals are not being provided in a bio-available form (i.e. a form which the horse can easily utilise within his body).

A horse on an inappropriate diet will show some or all of the following characteristics, depending on how bad the dietary imbalance has become:

- Loss of performance, sluggishness.

- Sole sensitivity: 'footiness' on hard or uneven ground.

- Flat feet or lack of concavity in the hoof capsule.

- Ripples or 'growth rings' in the hoof capsule.

- Stretched white line in the dorsal wall.

- Deviation in angle of growth: a 'bell-shaped' hoof capsule.

- Acute lameness owing to laminitis.

- Shifting weight from foot to foot, usually on the forefeet.

These problems can be progressive – a horse who is laminitic will show early warning signs by becoming mildly 'footy' on hard ground before the laminitic attack makes him acutely lame. Similarly, a horse may have ripples in his hoof walls, stretched white lines or flat feet, without ever reaching the stage of clinical laminitis.

The earlier the problem is caught (and the fewer the number of times the horse has been exposed to it) the less damage will be done to the hoof, and the quicker the problem can be reversed.

Of course, if you have any suspicion that your horse has laminitis, your first call must be to your vet, but if your horse is showing one of the more minor problems, then a change to his diet may be all that is required.

What about shod horses?

Notice how many of the characteristics of inappropriate diet directly affect the hooves! They affect shod hooves too and, of course, diet is just as important for a shod horse, but in a shod horse, unlike a barefoot horse, you will not see the effects so early.

The problems will still be there (how many shod horses are 'footy' when they lose a shoe?) but you will not necessarily be so aware of them. Peripheral loading with a shoe physically raises the sole from the ground, which means that the earliest warning signs of sole sensitivity on challenging surfaces may not be apparent.

Optimising diet

So, if you want to optimise the condition of your horse's hooves, you need to optimise his diet – but what does this mean in practice?

One of the biggest challenges in the UK is the climate – it's one of the reasons why barefoot performance horses remain less common here than in the US, or Australia.

Sensible owners all want our horses to live in a natural environment and to eat a natural diet. In the UK, traditionally the closest we come to being able to provide a 'natural' environment is to turn our horses out in fields to eat grass.

Turnout in a field certainly allows our horses to move more, and express more natural behaviour, than when they are kept stabled. It also provides 24/7 forage, which is much closer to 'natural' feeding than the restricted amounts of hay that are often fed to stabled horses. However, it can come as a surprise to realise that turnout on grass is often far from ideal for creating perfect hooves.

We've already highlighted how horses with excellent hooves tend to roam around vast areas and browse freely on many varieties of forage. Superficially, turnout in a field appears to mimic a natural diet – but the reality can be quite different.

The UK's wet weather and mild temperatures mean that grasses grow extremely well here. Add to that the effects of cultivation and one starts to realise that an artificially fertilised field, which has been seeded with a monoculture, or single species, such as ryegrass, is not ideal.

However, even in old, permanent pasture there is less biodiversity than there would be in an uncultivated area. Our fields have fewer species of grasses and significantly fewer other plants (such as shrubs and sedges) than there would be in the thousands of acres that are available to feral horses.

Cultivation not only limits the plant diversity, but the very species which thrive in the UK's fields are usually those grasses which are higher in non-structural carbohydrates and lower in fibre. Remember that the horse evolved to eat lots of low-quality, low-fructan, high-fibre plants, and you can see that a lovely green British field, in April or May, is roughly the nutritional equivalent to a year's supply of chocolate-covered doughnuts for us!

It might be all right if our horses ate less when the grass was richer, but their genetic switch is set to eat for 17+ hours a day. Like an office worker in a sedentary job who still eats three square meals a day, our horses carry on eating as their genes tell them to, even when they already have more than enough calories on board.

To compound the problem, horses are 'trickle feeders'. Unlike humans, they need an almost constant throughput of large amounts of fibre to maintain proper gut function.

Although lush, green grass is high in fructans and protein, it does not contain proportionally very much fibre, compared to the coarse, stemmy forage the horse evolved to eat. On high-sugar, low-fibre pasture, the horse has to eat much more grass in order to have enough fibre in his system and this sweet grass is highly palatable, encouraging the horse to gorge. This leads to the double-whammy of a horse on this type of grazing consuming far more sugar, fructans and protein than he needs, simply in order to get enough fibre.

This dangerous double-whammy can also occur on short, stressed grass – ironically the sort of grazing often found in 'starvation paddocks'. Like lush pasture, this type of grazing is low in fibre and high in fructans.

In an ideal world, what should our horses be eating? Desert grazing is more natural – it is high in fibre and low in sugars – but can we also find this more natural type of forage even in the much wetter environment of the UK?

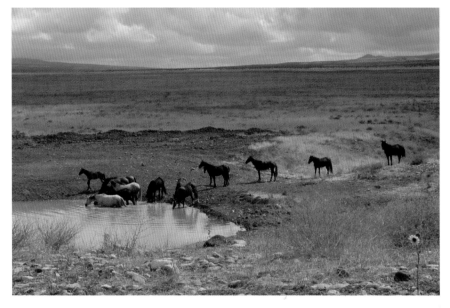

Mustangs in a desert environment.

The Exmoor ponies in the photo on page 90 live in an area of high rain-fall and almost constant moisture, and yet they have excellent hooves because they live on rough moorland rather than on rich pasture. The Exmoor is a very primitive breed, which researchers have shown to be genetically unique. Although these ponies live in a wet UK climate they live on rocky terrain and eat a diet with great variety, including herbs, shrubs and a huge range of moorland plants and grasses. They roam over many thousands of acres browsing, much as their ancestors will have done. Their high-fibre, low-sugar, high-mileage lifestyle is perfectly suited to developing healthy hooves. Interestingly, but perhaps not surprisingly, once these ponies leave the moor and their feral lifestyle, they become prone to obesity and laminitis.

In practice, of course, most of us don't own hardy Exmoor ponies and we don't have thousands of moorland acres available for turnout. So if grass is so problematical, what *can* we feed our horses if we want them to have the best possible hooves?

Feral Exmoor ponies.

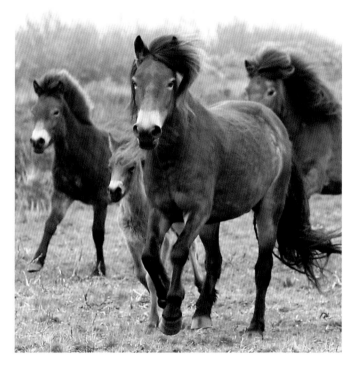

A breakthrough

We know from our observations (quite literally!) in the field, that grass has a radically different effect on horses' hooves compared to hay or haylage. A horse who will become 'footy' when turned out to graze ad lib on summer pasture will remain sound on challenging surfaces when fed ad-lib hay or haylage made from the same pasture.

For a long time, this puzzled us, and we struggled to work out what was the nutritional difference between the grass and the preserved forage – this had to be the key to the problem. It's hard to measure *precisely* what the difference is, because when the nutritional content of grass is measured, it is usually on a dry matter basis. And dried grass is, of course, virtually indistinguishable from hay. In addition, hay or haylage is usually made from mature, tall-stemmed grass whereas, when grazing, horses crop mostly short, young grass.

The exception is when grass is flash-dried. Interestingly, unlike hay or haylage, flash-dried grass products can cause similar problems in hooves to fresh, green grass. The difference is that flash-drying is known to preserve the fructan levels; by contrast when grass is preserved as hay or haylage, fructan levels start to drop soon after grass is cut (and are further reduced in haylage by fermentation). Suddenly everything makes sense!

Practical advice on forage

- Restrict access to fresh grass, especially at times when fructan levels are high and mineral levels are low.

- Fructan levels in grass are highest in spring and summer, and are also higher during the day and after a frost, so avoid these times if you can.

- Fructans are higher in short, stressed grass, and fibre is lower, so tall, stemmy grass is often safer. Quantities should still be monitored carefully and grazing restricted if necessary.

- If your horse does not tolerate grass well, you are not alone! Very few horses will have healthy hooves once turned out on unlimited UK spring grass. Meadow haylage and meadow hay are much lower in fructans, and can be given to most horses ad lib. If the non-structural carbohydrate ratio is more than 10 per cent (which can be determined by forage analysis), this can be reduced in hay by soaking.

- Haylage (provided it is made from mixed pasture, not single-species grass) is more palatable than hay, often has better mineral levels, and is better for the horse's respiratory system. It is lower in fibre than hay, so needs to be fed in larger quantities to provide enough fibre.

- If haylage is too rich for your horse and he is gaining too much weight or has a runny discharge when defecating, try a later cut or switch to hay. Hay often needs to be soaked for 10–30 minutes to reduce spores. Soaking hay for more than 30 minutes reduces its sugar content even further, but also leaches out other nutrients.

- Unlimited hay or haylage allows horses to trickle feed, and compared to grass, it is a low-sugar, high-fibre forage. This fulfils both physiological and behavioural needs, and you can also be sure that your horse is getting the fibre he needs without the high fructan levels which can lead to hoof problems.

- Grazing muzzles can occasionally be useful but, as a general rule, horses seem happier on a dry lot with ad lib hay or haylage than they do turned out to grass in a grazing muzzle. Muzzles can only be used for short periods, and severely restrict the amount of fibre a horse can eat. They can also be extremely frustrating for the horse and are prone to rubbing. Of course, if a muzzle breaks or comes off, the horse is then able to gorge.

- Try to avoid single-species forage, even as hay or haylage. Many dairy farms have turned to making their rich dairy grasses into haylage for horses. Beware this type of forage. Ryegrass in particular, a very common grass on dairy farms because of its high yield and high nutritional content, is high in non-structural carbohydrates. In any case, it's not natural for horses to eat monoculture, and they appreciate variety. Different plants also have different nutritional values, and a broad range of plants gives a more balanced diet.

- Every horse and every field is different. Nutritional values in grasses change season by season, day by day, hour by hour; equally forage that seems fine for one horse may not suit another. Your horse's hooves and his soundness will be the best indicator of whether his forage is suiting him or not, and these should always be your guide.

Supplementary feeding

For most horses, forage should form very much the major portion of their diets. For most horses, though, forage alone will not be enough, even if it provides enough calories and protein.

Providing additional feed for our horses is important, and there are two main reasons for doing this:

- To supply minerals, vitamins and trace elements, in which the diet would otherwise be deficient.

- To provide additional energy for horses who are working hard or need to gain weight.

We think it's worth spelling this out, because the horse-feed market is big business, and huge amounts of money are spent on advertising. We horse owners make great advertising targets, too, because we all want our horses to look and feel healthy, and it can be easy to lose sight of these two simple basics.

You don't need to become an expert in equine nutrition, but understanding the fundamental building blocks on which a horse's diet is based is extremely important. It's a bit like knowing enough to cook a balanced meal, rather than simply buying oven-ready dinners!

Vitamins, minerals and trace elements

Everything we feed our horses contains vitamins, minerals and trace elements. Horses in the wild receive no supplements, so why do we often need to add extra vitamins and minerals to our domestic horses' feeds? The reasons are as follows.

- The levels in forage will vary with the seasons, and as our horses often work all year round, they may need extra as levels in forage fall.

- Our feeds and forages are harvested from relatively few species; our fields are also cultivated so the wide range of herbs and plants which feral horses could browse to gain extra minerals are not available to our horses.

- Artificially fertilised soil, which is used to grow most non-organic forages and feeds, can be low in key minerals.

- Parts of the UK have known mineral deficiencies that require supplementation (and almost all forage lacks *some* minerals).

It sounds as if the ideal would be to find out what the mineral balance of our forage is, and we could then feed a bespoke supplement that just topped up anything that was missing.

In real life, though, its not always possible to have a full mineral analysis done, and even the most detailed analysis will only provide a rough guide, as mineral levels vary from one field to the next (except in intensively farmed monoculture crops) and from season to season.

Just to make things even more complicated, some horses also seem to need higher levels of minerals added to their diets than others, so in a group of horses kept on the same forage, some may be deficient in minerals while others are assimilating enough.

A lack of minerals can affect the whole horse, as can an excess. Minerals and vitamins work in balance with each other, and so the whole diet needs to be taken into account if you are providing a supplement. This can be very difficult, particularly with horses, as the majority of their diet should be forage which, as we've just seen, has fluctuating energy and mineral levels.

As it's so difficult to discover exactly what minerals our horses might already be getting in their diets, the easiest way to 'balance' a diet is often to add a broad-spectrum mineral supplement.

In practice, we find that if horses are provided with an appropriate high-fibre, low-sugar diet, and are given a bio-available, broad-spectrum mineral supplement, then over time they will often show some surprising improvements in condition or behaviour. They may become calmer, have a glossier coat or become less over-reactive. Very often, though, the biggest changes you will see will be in the hooves.

The hoof is a dynamic, living structure, and in a barefoot horse it is working hard. We have observed mineral deficiencies seriously affecting hooves, often causing sole sensitivity or loss of hoof wall connection.

There are lots of mineral supplements on the market. They are sold either as pelleted feed or as powders, but they often contain minerals in a form which horses may not be able to assimilate well – that is, in a 'pharmaceutical' form, divorced from organic matter. Since horses have evolved to digest plants, we believe that, if possible, it is best to feed them plant-based mineral supplements. These types of plant-based minerals can then be easily absorbed in the equine digestive system.

Research comparing mineral absorption levels has, in fact, shown that for some minerals, such as selenium, there is improved bio-availability when minerals are derived from plant sources rather than given in their inorganic form.

Even more compellingly, for us, there have been a number of horses on our own books who have shown improved hoof function when given plant-based supplements.

It is *always* worth reading feed labels! Many supplements have an impressive list of mineral levels, but when you read the ingredients list you may find that most of the minerals are not derived from plants but are added in their inorganic form (such as ground-up rock), which may not be as bio-available to the horse.

Similarly, if your horse is a barefoot horse, or is sensitive to sugars and cereals (most are!), then read the label to find out what the base ingredients of the supplement are. Many contain glucose, molasses, syrups and cereals in order to make the supplements more palatable. Even though the quantities are relatively small, they can be enough to make sensitive horses footsore.

We have found that a supplement based on linseed (giving omega 3 fatty acids, fat-soluble vitamins and copper), brewers' yeast (giving chromium, selenium and B-vitamins) and seaweed (giving a wide range of minerals and trace elements) provides a good balance of bio-available, essential minerals and can be used safely on most horses.

Table 2, at the end of this chapter, gives more information on recommended feeds.

Hooves and magnesium

Our observations of barefoot horses suggest that, as well as the minerals calcium, zinc, and copper, and the B-vitamin biotin, known to be important for hoof growth, magnesium and chromium levels in the diet are also crucial.

These minerals both play an important part in increasing insulin sensitivity, which is essential for regulating blood-glucose levels, as explained in greater detail later. Magnesium is also one of the key macro-minerals in the body, and works closely with calcium and phosphorus. Low levels of magnesium can impair muscle and nerve function, and circulation.

It's extremely common for horses who have been mineral-deficient to grow a better quality, more tightly connected hoof capsule once they have been fed a broad-spectrum mineral supplement and additional magnesium for at least six months.

So, can you tell whether a horse is deficient in magnesium? With some minerals, a blood test can show up whether a horse is deficient, but unfortunately this is not the case with magnesium, as blood-magnesium levels will normally be maintained even if other areas of the body are already low in magnesium. In humans, a serum test is used to determine magnesium levels, but this is not available for horses.

As a result, it is only after supplementing (in other words, if you see improvements in the actual hoof) that you can see evidence of whether the horse needed the additional magnesium. Fortunately, magnesium oxide is safe to supplement since an excess is not toxic and will be excreted by the horse.[14]

The vast majority of horses who receive additional magnesium show clear benefits to their hooves. In fact, all of the horses who have come to us for rehabilitation have shown improved hoof capsule quality and connection within two to three months. They also demonstrate improved hoof function after supplementation, so it does seem clear that many equine diets are low in magnesium.

It is certainly the case that magnesium deficiency is a well-known problem in other grazing animals in the UK, particularly cattle and sheep. It is a serious problem for farmers, especially in the spring when levels of magnesium in the grass fall. In many areas it is standard practice to give magnesium supplements to cattle and sheep.

In horses, this has not been done in the past, although there are a number of equine supplements available containing magnesium which are generally marketed as calmers.

Typically, these supplements are not only an extremely expensive way of providing magnesium, but also often contain poorly absorbed magnesium in extremely small quantities (2–5 g per day, again read the label!). In fact, we have found that (depending on the calcium levels in the horse's diet), performance horses can require up to 25 g of magnesium per day.

We started experimenting with magnesium supplementation a few years ago. Nic was trimming a group of horses at one yard who had been barefoot for some time, and had hooves that looked fine, but who were persistently footsore on stones. In passing, the yard owner mentioned that the fields these horses grazed were very low in magnesium, so in desperation Nic suggested that the owners talk to their feed company about adding magnesium.

Six weeks later she was amazed to see that the horses were able to march along a stony track in total comfort.

Since then we have found that many horses have less sole sensitivity and grow a tighter, better-connected hooves once they are given additional magnesium. Of course, if a horse already has enough magnesium in his diet, there will be no effect – and nor will magnesium-based calmers improve that horse's behaviour.

Magnesium works in balance with other minerals in the body, and the ratio of calcium to magnesium (which should be 2:1 in the diet)[15] is very important.

Magnesium deficiency can make horses hyper-alert, or spooky, and can also trigger muscular problems like tying up.

Magnesium is not only essential in balancing calcium levels (and vice versa) but, with chromium, it also has a key function in increasing sensitivity to insulin, the hormone that regulates blood-glucose levels.

Both human diabetic patients and insulin-resistant horses have typically low levels of magnesium, and we have seen some insulin-resistant horses benefit from magnesium supplementation.

We don't know exactly why magnesium deficiency can also cause hoof problems, although in humans, magnesium and chromium deficiency can cause problems with peripheral circulation and symptoms associated with adult-onset diabetes.[16] Maybe we are seeing a mild, long-term version of the same problem in horses with magnesium and chromium deficiencies. It has already been documented that in some cases insulin resistance in horses is a cause of laminitis.[17]

Lots of factors can combine to trigger magnesium deficiencies. Many fields and soils are inherently low in magnesium. Artificial fertiliser or incorrect soil pH levels can also reduce the uptake of magnesium by growing plants. If you compare soil and forage samples, and the forage shows low levels of magnesium but the soil levels are adequate, this is likely to be the problem. Plant growth rate may also be an issue: fast-growing spring grasses are high in fructans and have proportionally lower levels of magnesium available, both for horses and for cattle and sheep.

As a final straw, many horse's diets are high in calcium – for instance derived from alfalfa, sugar beet and cereals – but don't contain sufficient magnesium to maintain the important 2:1 ratio. These foods can cause availability to be reduced again, as high calcium levels also block magnesium uptake.

Because of the important interaction between calcium and magnesium, you should try to assess the approximate levels of calcium in your horse's diet before feeding additional magnesium (see Table 1).

It is also important to use a safe source of magnesium as a supplement. Unfortunately, magnesium is one of those minerals that is difficult to provide adequately through plant sources alone, so other sources have to be considered. Traditionally, Epsom salts (magnesium sulphate) were used, and are still found in some feeds today. However, this is not a good source of magnesium: although cheap, it actually has relatively low levels of magnesium (10–15 per cent), is poorly absorbed and can irritate the gut[18] and is best not given to horses.

Feed	Sugar beet (unmolassed)	Alfalfa	Oats	Grass hay (varies!)	Haylage (varies!)
Ca as %	0.91	1.47	0.11	0.47	0.56
Mg as %	0.23	0.29	0.16	0.18	0.20
Ratio	4:1	5:1	1:1.5	2.5:1	2.8:1

Table 1 Calcium and magnesium levels in some common feeds.

Magnesium salts are used in some liquid supplements, but these are extremely expensive and generally provide too little magnesium (as little as 2–3 grams per day). Some magnesium compounds (magnesium aspartate and glutamate) should be avoided because in humans they can be neurotoxic.[19]

A far better source is magnesium oxide, which is generally well tolerated. In its pure form it can be expensive, but agricultural, animal feed grade, calcined magnesite has good levels of magnesium oxide and is very cost-effective. It is not the best-absorbed form of magnesium, but it is widely available.

(Magnesium citrate contains a lower level of magnesium than magnesium oxide, but in a more bio-available form.[20] It is available in health food shops and is used in human supplementation, but it is not widely used in horses yet, although that may change.)

Provided you use magnesium oxide and balance the levels of calcium in the horse's diet, it is usually easy for the horse to excrete any excess as it is water-soluble.[21] A horse whose droppings become loose after being given additional magnesium may well already have enough in his diet, and so the supplementary magnesium should be reduced.

Some rough guidelines of calcium and magnesium levels in commonly used feeds are set out in Table 1, or you can seek specific advice from an independent equine nutritionist. Generally, you can see that calcium is over-supplied in comparison to magnesium, especially in alfalfa (lucerne) and sugar beet, and the ratio is much higher than the 2:1 ideal level.

Suggested amounts of various supplements are set out in Table 2 at the end of the chapter.

Notes on compound feeds

Recently, feed manufacturers have become aware that some of us are more interested in our horses' hooves than perhaps we used to be, and there are now lots of feeds and supplements which claim to improve your horse's hoof health. It is probably only a matter of time before one of them comes up with 'Barefoot' horse feed!

The problem with compound feeds is that, despite the labelling, they often contain ingredients like sugars, starches and chemicals that are not good for hooves. Frequently, they either have an inadequate level of minerals or only supply enough minerals when fed in large quantities, which owners are understandably reluctant to feed.

Although it is normally a legal requirement that ingredients and additives are listed, this is usually done in small print on an innocuous white label, which is frequently detached during transportation. By contrast, terms like 'low-sugar', 'ideal for laminitics', 'high-fibre' or 'totally natural' can be plastered in large, brightly coloured print on the bags, and have no legal definition. This type of marketing means that we don't always realise what we are actually feeding.

As with supplements, it is always important to read the ingredients list, not just the marketing blurb.

For instance, a well-known (and otherwise reputable) feed company sells one product which has emblazoned on the bag a promise that it is 'low in sugar, safe for laminitics'. Unfortunately it contains 10 per cent molasses, and we have seen a significant number of ponies who actually developed laminitis when they were fed the product, but were totally sound once it was removed from their diets and they were fed a genuinely low-sugar, high-fibre diet containing more bio-available minerals.

As well as sugar, which is often added to make feeds more palatable, most compound nuts and mixes also contain quantities of cereals, which are high in starch. As high levels of starch can compromise hoof and gut health (even causing laminitis in the most severe cases) it is worth avoiding these if you can.

Again, labelling can cause confusion. Many owners who would not dream of feeding their horses straight oats or barley are innocently giving their horses a couple of scoops of 'pasture mix' per day, thinking that because it is labelled 'for good-doers', 'non-heating' or 'for horses in light work' it does not contain cereal or starch. Yet when you read the ingredients list, rather than the marketing blurb, you will find that these mixes contain oats, wheat, barley, molasses and a host of other ingredients from which a horse in light work is highly unlikely to benefit.

Current advice is that if a horse is fed more than 0.2–0.4 per cent of his bodyweight per meal as starch, there is a risk of overloading the caecum and large intestine.[22] Dr Chris Pollitt's research has shown that this type of starch overload can be a trigger for laminitis.

Most cereals (oats, barley, wheat, maize) are high in starch, ranging from about 45 per cent starch (oats) to over 70 per cent starch (maize). As there are plenty of other, safer ways of supplying horses with extra energy, we recommend that most horses are fed a low-starch, low-cereal diet, which will also benefit their hooves, whether they are barefoot or shod.

Hard-working horses

Of course, hard-working horses may need more than just hay or haylage, but fibre feeds (like alfalfa) or high-oil feeds can supply as much if not more energy than cereals, in a form that is safer for both gut and therefore hooves. Oil-rich feeds added to a horse's diet can be a useful source of slow-release, long-term energy, which avoids the risks of making horses over-excitable but leaves them equally forward-going.

Adding these feeds avoids the dangers of high levels of starches associated with cereals and, as with many feeds, oil-rich feeds are safest and most effective when they are fed in the least processed, least refined form. Refined oils are high in fat but often low in other nutrients, whereas whole oil feeds, like linseed or coconut meal, have a better amino-acid profile and still contain fat-soluble vitamins and minerals.

Oils are also a valuable source of omega fatty acids, and omega 3 in particular can have an anti-inflammatory effect. In our opinion linseed is the best source of omega 3 for horses.

It goes without saying (we hope!) that since horses are natural herbivores, it is generally not a good idea to feed them animal fats, such as fish oils.

We have suggested some practical diets for horses working in the toughest disciplines (racing, eventing, hunting, endurance) Table 2 at the end of this chapter. We have used these ourselves and recommended them to clients for several years. We know they are not only effective but also safe for hooves.

Ingested substances that might cause harm

Wormers

UKNHCP trimmers and farriers started reporting sole sensitivity following worming some years ago. This can frequently occur in previously sound barefoot horses, and is especially common when combination wormers are used. These are designed to tackle several types of worm in a single dose, and although convenient for owners, mean that the horse is exposed to a double dose of toxins.

Many of the new generation combination wormers are also long acting. In reality this means that the active ingredients are stored in the horse's body, in the fat, so that they remain active for up to three months. This seems convenient for us and makes it appear as if it is better for the horse (as wormers are administered less frequently over a yearly cycle). However, if a horse were to have a reaction to such a wormer it could take months for the effects to subside.

A previously healthy yearling suffered acute sole sensitivity and the laminar connection in his hoof capsules was seriously damaged immediately after he was treated with a combination wormer. Perhaps it was simply coincidence, but his owner has since changed her worming programme.

As a rule, along with many veterinary practices, we now recommend that owners use faecal egg counts and blood tests for tapeworm, to determine whether there is a need, before using chemical wormers. If chemical wormers have to be used, we would advise that only a single-action dose is used at any one time.

After ingesting a long-acting combination wormer one horse (who had previously been sound over all surfaces barefoot) took only forty-eight hours to become so 'footy' that he was lame on hard surfaces. After four days he was lame on soft surfaces too. It took three months for his hooves to return to being able to traverse challenging surfaces again. Although this was a severe reaction we have seen other occasions when wormers have made competent barefoot horses 'footy' over challenging surfaces.

Mycotoxins

Mycotoxins are fungal poisons that grow on a range of plants, both grasses and cereals. In humans and other animals, mycotoxins are known to be responsible for a range of diseases, and for non-specific symptoms like poor growth or poor appetite.

One variety of mycotoxin, ergot, is known to cause neurological, reproductive and vascular problems in many animals, including horses.

We became interested in mycotoxin poisoning after a client, whose horses all developed severe insulin resistance, found that her paddocks and hay crop were contaminated by ergot. Since then, we have seen other cases where insulin-resistant horses were being fed forage contaminated by ergot.

These horses all have recurrent moderate to severe laminitis, despite a low-starch, low-sugar diet, and they also show raised cortisol and glucose levels.

In humans, ergot poisoning can lead to a range of symptoms including damage to peripheral circulation.

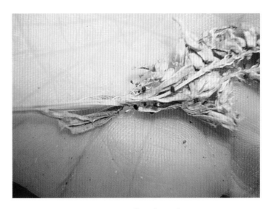

Ergot on hay.

Since these horses are known to have ingested low levels of ergot over a prolonged period, it is possible, although unproved at the moment, that ergot poisoning is a contributory factor in their insulin resistance.

A number of vets have reported more cases of insulin resistance in horses over the last few years, which may be a result of improved testing. However, since ergot flourishes in damp weather, we wonder whether ergot, or other mycotoxins, are also increasing as a consequence of the UK's recent wet, mild winters and damp, humid summers.

Additionally, in recent summers, hay and haylage has been difficult to make well, in some areas, and harvesting has sometimes had to be done in less than ideal weather conditions. This provides opportunities for mycotoxins to flourish.

Unfortunately at the moment there are no widely available testing facilities in the UK where forage can be checked for mycotoxin contamination, although it can be done in the US.

More research is needed into whether there is a link between horses ingesting this type of toxin and, over time, the cumulative effects contributing to insulin resistance.

Contaminated water

Don't forget that water quality can have a profound effect on health. Water is the nutrient needed in the greatest quantity. A healthy horse will drink around 5 per cent of his bodyweight of water per day, with this percentage increasing following work, in hot conditions, or if associated with a dry (e.g. hay-based) diet. A 500 kg (1,100 lb) horse will therefore drink 25+ litres (about 40 pints) of water a day, depending upon conditions.

Horses who drink from streams and ponds can have their water contaminated by agricultural run-off (for example, from artificially fertilised fields) or by rubbish which has been dumped and leached into the water.

If your own drinking water needs to be treated in order to maintain its

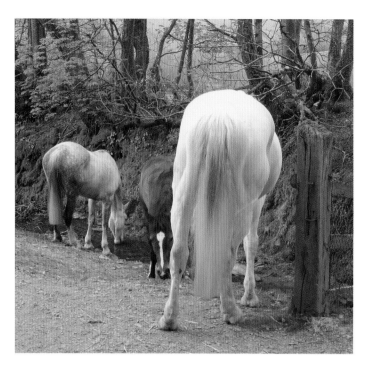

Horse drinking from a natural source.

quality, then it may be that your horse's water needs to be checked as well. Certainly it is worth either testing the water, or providing horses with water from another source if they only have access to a natural water supply and do not seem to be thriving.

Dietary summary

- Use Table 2 at the end of the chapter as a guide to safe feeds. All the feeds listed have been tried and tested over a number of years by barefoot horses in many disciplines.

  We've included a wide range of feeds, so you should able to find something that will suit your horse, whether he is a retired good-doer who needs to keep his weight down, or a lean, fussy Thoroughbred who is hunting twice a week!

- If you have your own land, get a soil analysis done and have your forage analysed regularly – ideally annually. This will give you a broad picture of what mineral deficiencies you may be dealing with, and will also give nutrient values for your hay or haylage.

- If you don't have specific information on availability of minerals, you should generally supplement with a broad-spectrum vitamin and mineral supplement, plus magnesium, especially if your horse has sole sensitivity, ripples, a stretched white line or flat feet.

- Generally, a horse with poor hoof wall is lacking key minerals, and once supplements are given, hoof growth will improve.

- Calcium and magnesium should broadly be balanced to ensure a dietary ratio of 2:1.

- Blood tests will identify some mineral deficiencies, but cannot be used to test for magnesium deficiency.

- Magnesium oxide is a safe source of magnesium, but do not use Epsom salts (magnesium sulphate) as a long-term additive as this can irritate the gut and only provides low levels of poorly absorbed magnesium.

- Don't feed cereals and starches, except in strictly limited amounts. Even a horse which is covering 65+ km (40+ miles) per week at speed will have more energy on a low-starch, low-sugar, high-fibre, oil-rich diet.

- Avoid high-sugar feeds. Check for molasses, glucose, dextrose, fructose and syrups on the labels of feed bags. Even those advertised as being suitable for laminitics may contain some or all of these ingredients. All are commonly added to feed to make them palatable, and amount to junk food for horses.

- Often, a horse who has been on a high-sugar, molassed feed diet will initially turn his nose up at a bucket of 'health food' which has no added sugar. Like toddlers, most horses need time to get used to new tastes, so keep presenting the new food (without offering a sugary alternative!). By the fourth or fifth day, your horse should have become accustomed to the taste, and long term (like us) most seem to feel better when they eat more healthily.

- Listen to the horse – if a horse is not improving, or a previously sound horse becomes 'footy', assess the diet first, as this is one of the most common causes of foot problems.

- In a horse who is not improving on a good diet, blood tests for insulin resistance, liver function and levels of some minerals (copper, zinc, selenium) and B-vitamins, can be useful.

- Be suspicious of free-flowing chaffs. As well as being an expensive way to feed forage, these can cause problems for some sensitive horses, even when they contain only 'safe' ingredients. It is not clear what the trigger is, although mould-inhibiting chemicals may be a problem. In a 'footy' horse it is always worth eliminating these feeds and monitoring for improvement.

- Use chemical wormers sparingly. Some horses are particularly sensitive to wormers. Worming with single-ingredient chemical wormers or using a natural wormer is much safer. Combining this approach with regular worm counts (and blood tests for tapeworm) will give a picture of an individual horse's worm burden and in some circumstances your chemical worming programme can be reduced or even stopped altogether.

- Take care with natural watering points as they can be susceptible to pollution. Providing an alternative water supply in addition to a stream or pond allows the horse more choice.

Problem-solving

Typically, if an otherwise healthy horse suffers from a dietary overload (for instance after being turned out on grass which is high in sugars) then it is possible to reverse the damage fairly quickly. The story of Morris, earlier this chapter, is a typical example: within a few days of being taken off the grass, the horse's system will readjust and the horse should be capable of working as normal.

Of course, the quicker the problem is spotted, the less damage will be done. This is one of the reasons why barefoot works best with hard-working horses. If you are working a horse regularly, you develop a feel for that horse, and can spot any deterioration in his soundness very early.

Initially, it may be nothing more than a gut feeling that the horse is not quite 100 per cent, or a suspicion that perhaps he is not quite as oblivious to challenging surfaces as he used to be. If you are able to take action at this stage, then usually no damage is done.

The exception is when a sensitive horse has been exposed to a chemical, such as a long-acting combination wormer. Because the active ingredients in these types of wormer are stored in the body for many weeks, it can take much longer – sometimes three months – for the horse to recover. Unlike with a dietary overload, if a horse has a bad reaction to a wormer there is no real remedy apart from time. It also appears that, after one exposure, the horse may be more sensitive if he is exposed to the same toxin again in the future.

- Note: In **Table 2** items in bold italics provide *essential minerals*, and (unless you are sure that all your forage is perfectly balanced) *should form part of the diet even when no additional energy or protein is required.*

Feed	Use	Supplier
Seaweed 50–100 g	Broad-spectrum minerals	Equus Health: Winter glow, summer shine Equimore No. 1
Brewers' yeast 25–100 g	Chromium, B-vitamins Selenium	Charnwood Milling
Linseed (cooked) 100–500 g	Omega 3, protein, copper High in oil Fantastic for coats and condition Facilitates absorption of other minerals	
Magnesium oxide (we are investigating more bio-available sources)	Should be balanced with calcium in 2:1 ratio Feed up to 25 g Mg per day (typically 50 g Calmag/MgO) if you are feeding high quantities of alfalfa and sugar beet or other high calcium forage Important for feet, brain, gut, muscles – one of the key minerals	Calcined magnesite (85% MgO) from agricultural feed stores Pure MgO from pharmaceutical wholesalers
Unmolassed alfalfa	Protein, variety of minerals High in calcium Feed no more than 1% bodyweight per day Good for horses in moderate/hard work	Dengie alfalfa pellets Charnwood Milling
Unmolassed sugar beet	Slow-release energy Highly palatable, relatively high-energy Ideal for good doers: gives bulk but is low in calories if fed in small quantities	Speedibeet Easibeet
Coconut meal	High in oil: 8–10% Low in starch Good source of protein, copper, magnesium Low in calcium Highly palatable Best for horses in hard work or needing extra condition May not suit insulin-resistant horses	Boomerang: Coolstance
Grass nuts	Energy, protein Don't feed to horses prone to laminitis/ sole sensitivity	Any feed merchant
Crushed oats	Energy – carbohydrate based Feed no more than 0.5% bodyweight per day (i.e. 2.5 kg/5½ lb max for a 500 kg/1,100 lb horse), split into at least 2 meals	Any feed merchant

Table 2 Dietary sources of various nutrients.

Feeds to avoid	
Molassed feeds and supplements	Always check labels, even on 'low-sugar' products
Flash-dried forages	Often high in fructans, especially grasses
Bagged chaffs	'Free-flowing' chaffs are often treated with mould-inhibiting chemicals
Single-ingredient mineral supplements (e.g. biotin, magnesium calmers), Also vitamin E supplements	Fine if recommended by an independent nutritionist or vet: in other cases, supplementing one mineral on its own can unbalance a diet
Animal products (e.g. fish oils)	Horses are vegetarians!

Table 3 Feeds best avoided.

8

Exercise and environment for the healthiest hooves

The commonplace that the horse is perfectly adapted for running should probably be modified…In fact the need to cover vast distances in search of food and water was most likely the crucial factor in its biomechanical evolution.

Stephen Budiansky, *The Nature of Horses*, 1997.

Horses evolved to move – lots! Exercise and environment are as crucial as diet for building great hooves because hooves grow in response to stimulus. The more work hooves do, the faster they grow and the stronger they become.

As well as growing faster, hooves that are working hard have improved circulation and proprioception. Working hooves also respond to pressure and stimulus to develop stronger, more resilient internal structures.

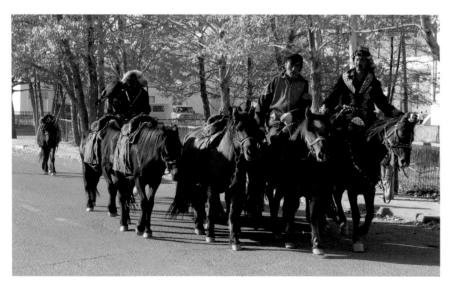

Horses in Mongolia working on the road.

In fact, hooves require work in order to develop properly, and this is especially true for the back of the foot. Robust structures at the back of the foot are essential. The hoof needs a well-developed digital cushion and lateral cartilages, with good vascularisation. To work effectively with good biomechanical function it should have strong frogs and heels. If a horse is weak in these areas, other parts of the foot, such as the laminae and pedal bone, will be put under inappropriate strain and the horse will be less comfortable and less capable.

Work is therefore one of the best ways to improve overall hoof performance, but it has to be the right sort of work.

The 'couch potato' factor

In a feral environment, horses have to cover many miles in order to find and consume enough forage. By contrast, in a domestic situation, horses only have to take a few steps in order to eat all day long. Turned out in a British field, their hooves get little stimulation from the soft, damp ground and over a few hours of grazing on green grass they will consume far more energy than they actually need. Of course once horses are stabled, their movement is even more restricted.

For comparison, feral desert horses need to roam around 40 km (25 miles) a day, on abrasive terrain, to find what they need to eat; feral Exmoor ponies on moorland move only about 5 km (3 miles) per day, on generally softer terrain, and domesticated horses in a field will move less than half that – only about 2.5 km (1½ miles) per day.[23]

The more distance a horse covers, the more he stimulates his feet. We have already seen that hooves respond to stimulus by increasing their growth rate, and harder-working hooves are generally healthier hooves as well.

Barefoot necessities

So, if we want to work our barefoot horses on all terrain in all disciplines we need their hooves to be capable of a higher daily mileage – nearer the sort of distance a feral desert horse would cover. In the endurance discipline, of course, horses are asked to perform over much greater distances on competition days, but if a horse's hooves are capable of covering 40 km (25 miles) day in, day out, they will normally produce hoof growth which is more than adequate for any discipline.

To get to this level of fitness, the hoof, like any other part of the body, needs training and preparation. If you enter for a marathon, or you plan for your horse to compete in eventing or endurance, you expect to put in months of training to get to the necessary fitness level. A horse's hoof is no different – we have already learned how hooves take years to strengthen and develop fully. As with the horse's musculature, good hooves are a product of time, correct work and stimulus.

Exercise is also essential if horses are to digest and use sugars in the diet effectively. Research has shown that insulin-resistant horses who are worked regularly have improved blood-glucose levels,[24] and we have seen in our own practices that insulin-resistant horses, like other horses, benefit enormously from moving more miles each day.

Lucy, an insulin-resistant pony, had been confined to a small area, half of which was bark, the other half concrete. This enabled her owners to ensure that she received lots of forage, but no grass, which was essential for her in order to avoid laminitis. She had daily driving exercise in a cart around the local lanes but needed front boots to protect her very damaged hooves. Then, over one winter, she was turned out into an area of hard tracks and farm buildings with another horse for company, and was able to roam over much larger distances. Within a matter of weeks the performance of her hooves had improved dramatically and several months later her improvement was such that she was happy pulling her cart without front boots.

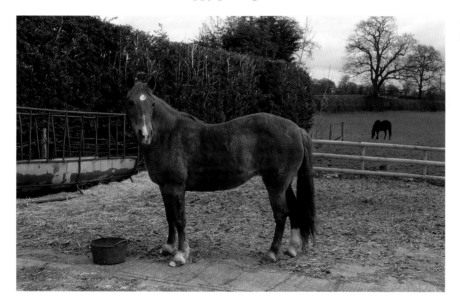

Lucy in her bark and concrete environment.

Movement as therapy

If a horse has basically healthy hooves, then it is relatively easy to bring hooves to full fitness.

With a horse who has previously been shod, or with a horse with poorly developed unshod hooves, some of the structures of the hoof may have atrophied or failed to develop and the horse may even be lame.

When a horse has suffered from a dietary or metabolic problem, the whole hoof capsule may be compromised. In these situations, movement will help to stimulate, strengthen and rebuild the weak areas of the hoof, and a correct diet will allow the hoof to build a better connection. The stimulus of movement will also speed up the growth of a new and better-attached hoof capsule. However, in order for movement to be therapeutic, it must be correct for that horse.

In practice, this means that the horse needs to be comfortable to land heel-first. If he cannot do this, then he is simply perpetuating bad biomechanics, and may even be causing more damage to soft tissue, such as muscle and tendons.

The combination of stronger structure and better hoof wall attachment will result in a more robust hoof, better able to perform.

The conditioning myth

Once a horse is comfortable on conformable surfaces*– on pea gravel, in fields or in the arena – the next challenge is to stimulate hooves on tougher terrain.

Work on more challenging ground is necessary in order to stimulate the hoof to grow more quickly, and in order to strengthen the internal structures of the hoof.

It is certainly therapeutic for a hoof to be working on tougher surfaces, and it is an important part of the fitness plan for any barefoot horse, but if you plan to work a horse extensively on hard surfaces such as roads, you need to increase the mileage steadily, to give the hooves the chance to increase hoof growth to match wear.

Both our own horses and those horses who are with us for rehabilitation live on varied surfaces. These surfaces include gravel, rock, concrete and earth, and as a result they cope happily with these surfaces when they are out and about.

Conversely, if your horse spends the majority of his time living on only a soft, supportive surface, you will need to build in lots of controlled exercise on a tougher surface if you want to be able to hack and compete on all terrain.

Be careful, though! A horse's capability over a tough surface will *not* improve simply because of increased exposure to that surface. It is never productive or fair to force a horse to work on a surface that he finds uncomfortable, and it is a myth that a horse who is uncomfortable on a surface needs repeated exposure to that surface in order to become sounder.

---

* A conformable surface is one which supports and loads the whole foot evenly. Rounded 5–10 mm gravel is typically used, and is an extremely comfortable surface even for horses with severely damaged hooves.

A conformable surface of pea gravel.

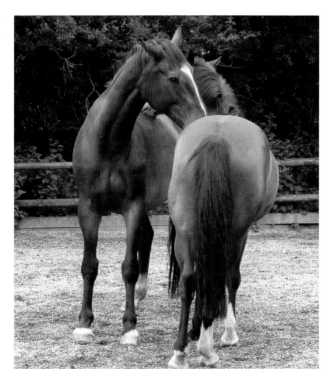

It is usually very clear from the horse's movement whether he is able to work on a tough surface or not, and a horse *must* be comfortable on a surface before you can usefully increase his exposure to it. In reality, repeated exposure *before* the horse is comfortable will only make him sore.

The 'conditioning myth' is very pervasive in some barefoot circles, so let's spell it out: working a horse when his feet are uncomfortable risks making him miserable, injuring him and damaging his trust in you. We have never seen a horse who is 'footy' on stones get better as a result of being ridden over stones. This is where it is essential that you are able to listen to your horse and analyse his capability.

Usually, the best way to improve sole sensitivity is to change the horse's diet. Even relatively simple changes (such as replacing grass with haylage or hay and boosting mineral levels) will frequently be enough to enhance hoof performance and comfort significantly.

Coming out of shoes

A horse with weak hooves is likely to need to develop and strengthen several structures in the hoof before he is truly capable of barefoot performance.

When we are asked to take a horse out of shoes, we will always assess his diet, hoof health and biomechanics first.

Working barefoot requires a horse to use his hooves in a different way:

he needs to be able to load the frog, sole and walls together. This is not something which happens with a shod hoof, as the shoe loads the periphery of the hoof.

Out of shoes, the hoof may breakover in a different place and the back of the hoof will play a more active role. This area of the hoof, instead of being restricted, will need to develop in order to be able to load and to be able to absorb shock, expand and contract.

Developing from an unhealthy or compromised hoof to a healthy hoof can put an enormous strain on the horse, so it is of paramount importance that we keep the horse comfortable as we allow him to strengthen and improve his hooves.

Practical steps

If the horse is sound in shoes and moving correctly, then we will ask the owner to make any necessary dietary changes for at least six to eight weeks before the horse comes out of shoes. By eliminating sole sensitivity through a correct diet, we find that most horses who were sound in shoes are comfortable and able to work from the day their shoes come off.

The sound horse

If the horse is sound and in work, and has been landing heel-first in shoes, we know that his biomechanics are not badly compromised.

Such a horse should have a frog and digital cushion which are in reasonable health, and which should start to improve very quickly. This horse would normally be comfortable to resume his current work levels in an arena or on grass straight away. Roadwork would also continue, but the distance would be built up over a few weeks, to allow the hoof time to respond by increasing horn production.

Depending on the strength of the frog and digital cushion, the horse might not be totally comfortable on stony, uneven ground, but he will not do himself any harm if he is allowed to pick his way over stones for a short distance. However, if you need to work the horse extensively on this type of surface within the first few weeks, the horse's welfare will require you to protect his hooves with boots.

The horse with compromised hooves

Very often it is not the sound horses but the lame ones whom we are asked to take out of shoes – usually because there are no other options left.

These horses may have poor-quality, cracked or crumbly hoof wall, thin soles and weak, under-run heels. Typically they are unable to land heel-first and, because of their compromised biomechanics, they often have internal soft tissue damage (for example to the deep digital flexor tendon or navicular bursa).

Generally this has gone hand-in-hand with a diet which has not supported good hoof wall connection, resulting in sole sensitivity, stretched white line, long dorsal wall or flat feet.

Again, the first thing to do for these horses is to ensure that their diet is changed to alleviate these problems. If a horse is weak in the back of the foot, the last thing he needs is for his soles to be sore as well, giving him nothing to stand on.

Our aim is to improve, develop and strengthen all these weak areas, but it can only be done over a period of weeks or months when the horse is able to move comfortably.

Once the diet has been improved, sole sensitivity will be reduced or eliminated. After about three months on this diet the hoof will show a dorsal hoof wall with an improved angle of growth from the coronet. This shows that the 'new' hoof capsule has a stronger laminar bond to the internal structures; over four to six months, as the new angle grows down, this will suspend the pedal bone higher within the hoof capsule and allow the sole to thicken, protecting the internal structures still more.

While this is happening, the horse will be able to resume work, but we must respect the fact that his hooves are weak.

We are now encouraging the horse to load centrally, instead of peripherally. This change will be stimulating weak structures. Normally, these horses will have been landing flat or toe-first, and as a result have atrophied or under-developed frogs, digital cushions and lateral cartilages. These structures will only develop in response to pressure and release so it is important to get them working. This is, however, a balancing act as it is essential not to overload them beyond their capabilities.

A horse who has been landing toe-first needs to spend plenty of time on conformable surfaces. Sand and pea gravel are excellent as they stimulate the sole, walls and frog but provide a broad weight-bearing surface. Work on grass will also usually be comfortable for the horse, and, like sand and pea gravel, encourages a heel-first landing.

Once the horse is comfortable on these surfaces, then short amounts of time on more challenging terrain is fine, provided it remains within the horse's comfort levels.

Maintaining the comfort zone

You need to listen to your horse just as you need to listen to your own body if you start a new exercise regime. If you go to the gym and overdo your first session, you will be stiff and sore afterwards, and may even be injured.

An effective exercise programme for hooves, as well as for us, needs to gradually and steadily increase work levels, while remaining within a safe and comfortable limit.

As a general rule, even horses with previously poor hooves will be capable of resuming a full range of work on supportive surfaces fairly quickly. They will usually be happy with roadwork within a few weeks, and roadwork is a useful way of stimulating hoof growth, so it should be a regular part of the horse's exercise programme if possible. Work on stony, uneven surfaces will normally be difficult for these horses, and it may be many months before they have developed sufficiently robust hooves to absorb shock on these surfaces.

Forelegs, hind legs

If horses have suffered from forelimb lameness in shoes, then once they are sound and able to resume work barefoot, we find that they sometimes appear to be short-striding behind for a short period, especially on circles or hard surfaces. This does not appear to be foot-related, and it is likely that this is a consequence of short-term muscle tension resulting from the horse's changed way of going. It passes quickly and can be avoided by working the horse on good ground and not performing tight turns.

In severe cases, very damaged hooves may never recuperate well enough to cope, and may always require protection in the form of shoes or hoof boots. This is rare, but can happen, particularly if the horse has been lame or moving incorrectly for a prolonged period.

Maximising movement; the concept of tracks

We've already seen that the traditional British way of managing horses is not ideal. Turnout in fields can cause dietary overload in the summer, and fields are often poached and sodden in winter. Stabling allows for more control of the horse's diet, but restricts movement and doesn't allow horses much opportunity for social behaviour.

If you've got a barefoot horse, you want his hooves to be rock-crunching all year round – but if you don't live in Arizona, and have to deal with green grass or torrential rain for most of the year (sometimes at the same time), what are the options?

The inspiration for tracks

For the last few years, we have kept our horses primarily on track systems. These were the inspiration of Jaime Jackson, who wrote a book in 2004 called *Paddock Paradise*.

His brilliant, but simple, idea was to create tracks round the edges of fields, rather than just turning horses out into the middle of them.

On a track, horses have more reason to move, as feed, water and shelter can all be placed in different areas. If you have several horses, they also encourage each other to move, as one of them goes off to investigate what might have changed round the corner, and the others follow.

Tracks are a relatively new idea, although they are rapidly becoming more popular. They are also a more effective way of managing fields than strip grazing or starvation paddocks, but, at their simplest, are no more expensive.

It is possible to devise a basic track with electric fencing, and this is very practical and can make minimal impact on the environment. Permanent fencing, however, is less nerve-racking if you find that electric fencing is prone to shorting out or that the battery sometimes runs out!

System	Advantages	Disadvantages
Field	Allows moderate movement Less work for owner Social environment for the horse	Rich grass in spring and summer Ground may poach in winter Hooves wet even in summer Can't use field for forage crop Shelter can be a problem Need to maintain fencing Requires 1+ acre per horse
Stable	Limits grass intake Horse protected from bad weather Can keep hooves dry Can use fields for forage crop Useful when space is limited	Restricts forage (usually) Restricts social behaviour Restricts movement Labour-intensive Cost of bedding Places hooves in an ammonia-rich environment
Track	Maximises movement Less work for owner than stabling Social environment for horse Keeps hooves drier than field Limited grass but ad lib forage Can use fields for forage crop Effective in small areas Avoids damage/poaching to fields, maintains plant biodiversity Varied surfaces allow for hoof stimulus	Need to maintain fencing Need to pick up droppings daily Track may poach in winter Surfaces can be costly to lay Requires investment of time and some creativity!

Table 4 Pros and cons of tracks.

Adapting your facilities

Creating a track is all about adapting your existing facilities, whether a livery yard, existing buildings or just a piece of land.

We've given some examples in the associated diagrams of how different facilities could provide track systems without the need to spend large amounts of time or money on the changes. One of the benefits of a track is that you need far less acreage than you would for turnout, so this can also be factored into your budget.

Track system for up to four horses

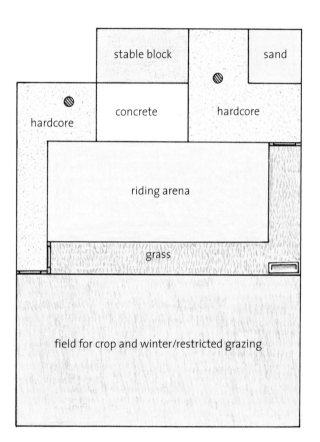

▭	Water
∿∿∿	Grass area which can be closed off in summer
▨	Hedge
▭	Gate
◉	Hay feeder
❀	Wooded area
⌇	Stream

Track system for up to eight horses

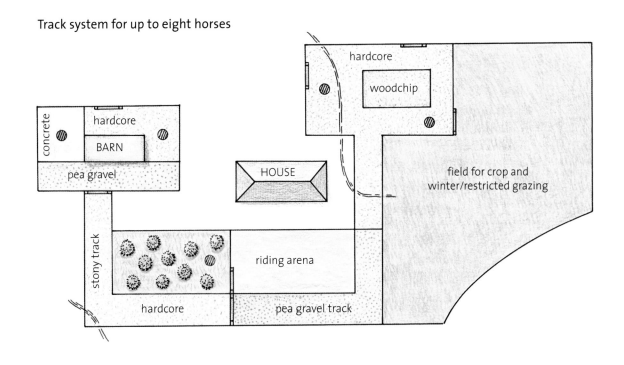

Alternative track system for up to eight horses

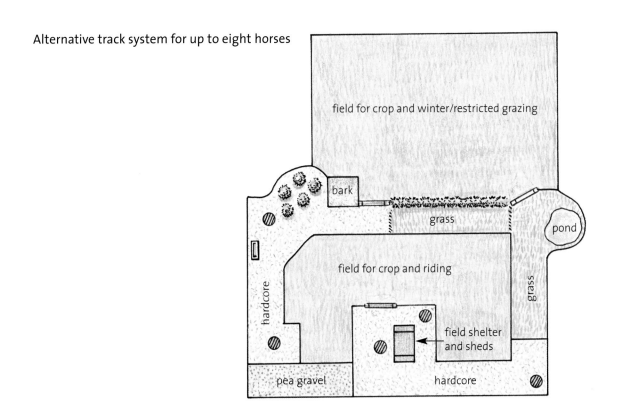

Practical advice on tracks

- Wet UK winters mean that tracks round fields may become poached unless they are very well drained. If putting in drainage is too expensive, then keep the track for spring and summer, and turn out on a bigger area in winter, when grass is less potent.

- If you want to be able to use your track system in winter, you may need to lay a hardcore base to improve drainage. Hardcore as a top surface will be too challenging for weak hooves, so you may need to top it up or create a path upon it with a more supportive surface.

- Pea gravel – rounded 5–10 mm (⅕–⅔ in) stone – or sand are comfortable surfaces for horses with poor hooves but should not be too deep; 10–15 cm (4–6 in) is usually enough. Both will last longer if they are laid over a membrane.

- Bark chippings are a cheap alternative to gravel or sand, but will rot away over a couple of years and can be trickier to muck out.

- Electric fencing is a quick and easy way to mark out a track, but needs to be checked regularly to avoid break-outs. This type of fencing can be made more robust by the addition of fence posts on corners and at regular intervals.

- Try to combine a track with existing facilities. For instance, a hardcore area that is used for parking could have a track running around the edge; an existing lean-to or field shelter can provide protection from the weather, and streams, ponds, hilly or wooded areas are all features that can all be incorporated to add variety.

- To maximise movement, spread out feeding stations and other essentials, like water and shelter, so horses have to roam to get what they need.

- If you have more than a few horses, make sure the tracks are wide enough for horses to get away from each other in case of bullying, and provide larger areas for them as well.

- Hay or haylage is best fed ad lib from cattle or sheep feeders, which allow horses to eat from ground level. 'Tombstone' feeders, or large, square feeders are ideal, as horses can't get their heads under the bars, but they can be expensive to buy new. We've successfully used round 'ring' feeders for years without a problem, but you should monitor your horses until they are accustomed to them. Round sheep feeders are lower than cattle feeders and thin plastic, like Clingfilm, should be wrapped right around the feeder to prevent hooves from getting in and hay from falling out.

- Hay or haylage will rot quickly once it gets wet, so either replenish it daily or feed it under cover.

- Have several feeding stations; this encourages movement and reduces the risk of bullying. If possible, have them in different locations so that, for instance, if there is a strong northerly wind horses can feed from a south-facing shelter, and vice versa.

- Horses who eat too much, or too fast, from big bale feeders can be slowed down by covering the feeders with netting.

9

Genetics and the healthiest hooves

We are all aware that different breeds of horse seem to have different hooves. Cobs, for instance, tend to have hoof wall of fantastic quality, which grows fast and is very robust. Their digital cushion and lateral cartilages usually remain strong even while shod. By contrast, Thoroughbreds are cited as having poor feet. Is this all down to genetics, or might there be other factors which are playing a part?

Genes are a constant throughout the horse's life, of course, and are a factor which we cannot alter in a living horse but, as we have said earlier, in our experience the majority of bad hooves are made, rather than born.

We have seen time and time again how, when given the opportunity, horses will grow better hooves. It seems that most horses are actually born with a blueprint for a good foot, and over their lifetimes they will continually try to grow the best possible hoof. However, as dietary and environmental factors intervene, the hoof is forced to adapt and many warp or deform.

In extreme circumstances, the original blueprint can become so marred that the horse can never recover a fully functioning hoof. However, the regenerative powers of the hoof are quite extraordinary and for most horses with 'bad' hooves, enormous improvements are possible.

Thoroughbreds are often cited as being a breed with genetically poor feet – a typical breed description we have seen reads: 'Thoroughbreds characteristically have flat feet'.

The owners of Dexter, the horse cited on pages 14–16, would have agreed with this description – their horse was lame and had been diagnosed with deep flexor tendonitis, often a precursor to navicular syndrome. His feet were shallow and under-run, with weak, crumbly hoof wall, but they assumed this was genetic.

After three months of rehabilitation, with a changed diet and an exercise programme designed to stimulate and support his hooves, there was a dramatic change in both the functionality and appearance of his hooves. His genes had not changed, but his hooves had – they were returning to the blueprint.

To confirm this, when you compare newly born Thoroughbred and feral foals, their feet simply don't show the differences that we associate with these breeds as adults. Thoroughbreds are not 'born' with bad feet; feral horses are not 'born' with good feet. Their feet are made, not bred.

10

Foot care for the healthiest hooves

The pros and cons of shoes

As stated earlier, we used to have our own horses shod, and recognise that, for many owners, shoeing is an attractive option, particularly if you have limited ability to control your horse's diet and environment.

Today the best shoeing uses as few nails as possible, so that the hoof capsule is allowed some expansion and contraction.

With Natural Balance shoeing, the frog is encouraged to engage, so as to stimulate the back of the foot and digital cushion, improving shock-absorption. The shoe is set back in order to encourage a heel-first landing. This puts less strain on tendons and ligaments. A Natural Balance shoe also allows the horse to breakover in a more natural way, unimpeded by a toe clip.

It is clear that these objectives are the same as those we are aiming for in a barefoot horse.

Drawbacks with shoeing

However, drawbacks exist with any shoeing system. The shoe is fixed for several weeks so, as the hoof grows, the horse's biomechanics are altered and, even if the shoe was perfectly placed on the day the horse was shod, a few weeks later it is likely to have migrated forward. In reality this means that the horse is likely to load the back of his hoof less the longer the shoe is on his hoof.

In addition, even with the best shoeing, the stimulus received by the frog is reduced, leading to a lack of development in the digital cushion and lateral cartilages. These structures are also restricted by the shoe, which reduces the perfusion available in the hoof. This in turn means that the foot is not able to absorb shock, or dissipate energy efficiently, and so greater concussive forces pass into the bones and soft tissue of the distal limb.

A final important difference is that, even with the most 'natural' shoe, the hoof is still peripherally loaded and restricted, so that the internal structures are not able to function as well as they would without a shoe. The way a Natural Balance shoe loads the front of the foot can also sometimes cause reduced circulation and stress to laminae.

Dr Bowker has hypothesised that the hoof functions best when it is loaded centrally. His research has shown that when a hoof is loaded peripherally, the density of the pedal bone will decrease over time – a similar effect to osteoporosis in people who do little weight-bearing exercise. The effects of this loading can be significant, with bones losing as much as 50 per cent of their density the longer they are loaded on their periphery.

Benefits of shoeing

If shoeing has these drawbacks, then why is it still such a popular option? There is no doubt that good shoeing can allow a horse's hoof to function beyond its current stage of development, and this can be extremely useful for owners in the short term.

For example, a horse who is showing sole sensitivity owing to a poor diet will appear much more comfortable once shod. Shoeing will not have solved the underlying problem, but it can be a practical way of alleviating the horse's discomfort.

The question of studs

Furthermore, a shoe allows you to use studs, which some riders view as essential when jumping. In fact, barefoot horses cope extremely well on all types of going without studs, and in many cases slip less than horses with shoes and studs.

It is possible that this is because a barefoot horse has better proprioception, and, like the human runner described in the section on Proprioception in Chapter 4, a better ability to adjust and compensate for different ground conditions.

There is also the possibility that studs do not actually work as effectively as we think they do. After all, on anything but the hardest possible ground, a 1.25 cm (½ in) of metal is not going to have sufficient leverage to significantly increase the traction of the hoof of a 500 kg (1,100 lb) horse galloping at more than 48 km (30 miles) per hour.

Paradoxically, studs undoubtedly have an effect on the hardest surfaces, like roads. Riders are consistently advised that leaving studs in when the horse is working on these surfaces is very unwise because of the jarring and imbalance they cause when they stabilise the hoof. Yet, when you think about it, these effects are a requirement if the stud is actually to do its job on any surface.

If studs are sufficiently stabilising to affect the footfall, a single stud will create a medial-lateral imbalance, as there will be a torque force as the stud lands but the limb continues to move for a fraction of a second.[25] If two studs are used, the limb will be more balanced, but again, if the studs are sufficiently stabilising to affect the footfall, any turns will cause strain on joints and ligaments.

Fortunately, once a horse is barefoot and balanced, he becomes extremely surefooted, and in fact most riders report that their horses slip less, rather than more, than they used to with studs.

Barefoot benefits

As we see time and time again, poor shoeing can lead to serious problems, and even good shoeing, if used too early in the horse's development, or for years without a break, can impair biomechanical function.

While horses with well-developed hooves that have been carefully shod can stay sound for many years, particularly on soft ground, other horses can be more quickly affected. This may be either because they have been poorly shod or because they are less able to compensate if their biomechanics are impaired.

Better biomechanics

We have found again and again by riding barefoot horses that the hoof functions more efficiently, and the horse moves more naturally, without a shoe. A shoe can provide a temporary boost in performance, but over time the hoof will gradually become less healthy. Peripherally loading the hoof contributes to the wasting away of the structures in the back of the foot, and the hoof is no longer able to maintain its internal health and integrity. Like putting a plaster cast on an arm, the rigidity of the shoe replaces developed internal structures and encourages them to atrophy.

For instance, if you break a bone in your hand, it will nowadays be put in plaster for no more than three to four weeks. Stabilising the bone for a longer time is great for the fracture, but means that ligaments, muscles and tendons become seriously compromised from lack of use and stimulus.

It certainly takes time for a barefoot horse to build hooves that can carry him over challenging surfaces, but once the horse has healthy hooves, there are no shoes that can match their superb biomechanics.

Fewer injuries

We know that injuries are reduced without shoes, particularly in horses whose conformation requires them to breakover off centre. Although still capable of inflicting serious damage, a horse who kicks without shoes on usually causes no more than a mild bruise, making it much safer to turn horses out in groups. This means that barefoot horses are also a safer option for owners, riders, vets and trimmers.

Surefootedness and shock-absorption

Proprioception and traction both improve without shoes. Horses are more aware of where their hooves are, and the terrain they are travelling over. This allows them to make constant compensations and adjustments for uneven or slippery ground. They also tend to absorb shock more efficiently than shod horses, partly because of their innate ability to adjust their gait to minimise impact, once they are aware of different surfaces.

In addition, the better internal function of a bare hoof (stronger digital cushion and lateral cartilages, greater proportion of fibro-cartilage and increased perfusion) enables the horse to dissipate energy within the hoof, rather than passing concussion into the lower limb.

Fringe benefits

We know that some horses seem to prefer not to be shod, perhaps because they find shoeing uncomfortable or painful, or because they have had bad experiences of shoeing in the past. It is not always clear exactly what they are objecting to, but these horses usually appreciate going barefoot. Most hoof care practitioners will have several horses on their books who needed to be sedated to be shod but behave angelically when they are trimmed.

Lastly we like the early warning that bare hooves give of dietary or metabolic problems. It can sometimes be a nuisance to have such good feedback, but it certainly makes you realise just how sensitive horses and their hooves can be! If you ride your horse barefoot you will feel any deterioration in his hoof performance straight away, and will often be able to resolve a minor dietary problem very quickly, before it becomes a major headache!

The 'barefoot trim'

Ironically, when people talk about 'barefoot' they often assume that it's all to do with trimming. We are constantly asked what sort of trim we do, and how it is different from a 'farrier trim' or a 'pasture trim'.

At a new yard, it will be the trimming that people want to watch, as if that is the key to barefoot performance. When people see dramatic changes in a hoof, they will ask how we have trimmed it, as though it is the trim that has made the changes in the hoof.

The truth is that you really can't improve a hoof *that* much by trimming it. If that sounds incredible, then let us explain.

In the photos adjacent is a hoof that has some serious problems. The back of the foot looks weak and the heels are under-run. To go with this, the toe is long, and the angle and rippling of the dorsal wall indicates that the laminar attachment is probably compromised. Sure enough, when you look at the solar view, the white line is stretched and the whole hoof lacks concavity and depth.

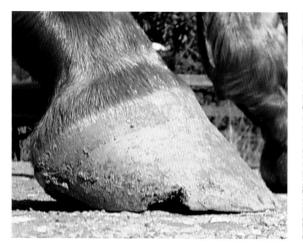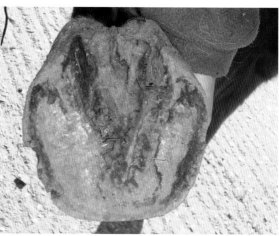

Two views of Dexter's foot in February, showing the problems detailed in the text.

The weak frog and contracted heels confirm that the digital cushion is poorly developed. This horse has been unable to use the back of his foot correctly for some time, and as a result not only has that area atrophied, but also there is resulting damage to the deep digital flexor tendon which has made the horse lame.

You could improve the mechanics of this foot by shortening the toe and bringing the breakover back. This would be an improvement, but on its own it will not be enough to strengthen the back of the foot or change the angle of the dorsal wall.

Shortening the toe would certainly force the horse to load the back of his foot more, but as the structures there are so weak, that might actually make him less sound. At best, the horse might start to engage the frog a little more, but even after trimming or shoeing, you will be left with a poorly attached hoof capsule, flat feet and collapsed heels.

A few weeks later, the hoof was beginning to change. There was a new angle of growth at the top of the dorsal wall, and a well-connected hoof capsule was starting to form. The new hoof wall growth was smooth and had no ripples, and once it had grown down the full length of the dorsal wall, the toe would be shorter and the breakover correct.

Six months after the original photos the hoof looked completely different. The following points are evident in the second pair of photos.

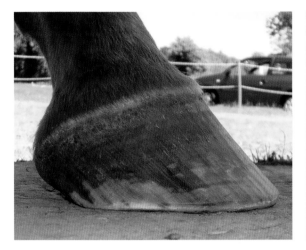 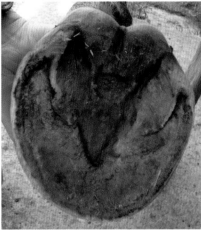

Dexter's foot 6 months after the previous pair of photos: now showing the improvements detailed in the text.

- The heel is now supporting the horse's weight, and the greater strength of the back of the foot demonstrates that the horse's biomechanics are much better. The lesion to the deep digital flexor tendon has healed and he is now landing heel-first. Of course he is much sounder, and in fact has been in full work, including fast work and jumping, for twelve weeks.

- The toe is shorter, with an improved breakover, and the dorsal wall has a consistent, well-connected angle.

- When you look at the bottom of the foot, the sole looks stronger and there is good concavity, indicating that the pedal bone is well-protected, suspended higher in the hoof capsule. The frog is healthy, and the heels are no longer contracted or collapsed.

Other factors supporting hoof health

It is important to understand that the changes just mentioned are *not principally* the result of a good trim. The improved connection between the internal structures and the outer hoof wall has come about because of a better diet. This diet is lower in sugars, higher in fibre and with an adequate level of bio-available minerals. This, not the trim, has led to a shorter toe, a well-protected pedal bone and thicker sole.

The development of the heels and frog has come about as a result of the horse living and working on a variety of conformable and challenging surfaces, which have provided support and stimulus. With the foot able to land heel-first, the frog has strengthened and the digital cushion is now able to do its job of absorbing concussion effectively.

As a better hoof capsule has grown in and the frog has developed, the heels have broadened and are no longer under-run.

Finally, with consistently improved biomechanics, the inflammation to the deep digital flexor tendon has gradually subsided and it has repaired.

The trim has supported and enhanced the mechanics of the new hoof as it has grown down by encouraging central loading of the hoof, but in the absence of correct diet and correct stimulus, even the best trim would not create a significantly better hoof.

Our 'pyramid' for a healthy hoof (see diagram) would look something like this:

Base: 65 per cent– diet – the foundation without which you can have nothing else.

Middle layer: 25 per cent – environment/exercise – the essentials to take hooves to the next level, and supported by correct diet.

Top layer: 10 per cent – trimming – 'the icing on the cake' (can make it look pretty, but is actually insubstantial in comparison to the founding layers).

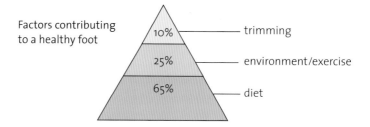

Factors contributing to a healthy foot — 10% trimming — 25% environment/exercise — 65% diet

Actually the concept is more like an iceberg than a pyramid – the trimming is the part you can see, but, like an iceberg, 90 per cent of the healthy hoof is the diet and environment that is out of sight.

If you are interested in improving hoof function or performance, the single most important thing you need to understand is how vital the underlying 90 per cent of this iceberg actually is. Any attempt to rectify a hoof using only a trimming or shoeing technique, and ignoring the rest of the iceberg, will be doomed to failure.

Any trimmer or farrier who tells you that what they do with their rasp is more important than what the owner does to manage the horse's diet and environment should be regarded with suspicion! It is extremely unlikely that the majority of the horses under this trimmer's or farrier's care will be romping over challenging surfaces, except in boots or shoes.

The dangers of trimming

The 'barefoot trim' has been elevated to an almost mystical status by some hoof care professionals, perhaps because they would like to believe that what they do is more beneficial to horse's hooves than is actually the case, or because they have not realised what a small part a trim plays in creating a truly healthy hoof.

However, the skill of the hoof care practitioner is vital, because it is certainly possible to lame a horse, either immediately or over time, with incorrect trimming.

Animal welfare organisations in the UK have expressed concern in recent years over one so-called 'barefoot' programme involving a technique which originated with a German vet called Strasser. The 'Strasser' method advocated aggressive trimming of the horse's sole and bars in some cases. The International League for the Protection of Horses (ILPH) has reported at least two successful prosecutions for animal cruelty after invasive trimming left horses seriously and persistently lame.

An enlightened approach to trimming

Fortunately, more enlightened farriers and trimmers were listening to the horses in their care and were determined to find ways of improving hooves which did not make horses sore.

A hallmark of the new approach was that trimmers tended to do less, rather than more, respecting the horse's natural movement. Their mantra was that horses should always be comfortable after they were trimmed.

One of the pioneers of this new approach was Pete Ramey, an American practitioner who started experimenting on his own horses. He found that by using what he termed the 'live sole' as a guide, and by observing how the horse wore his own feet, he could trim in a way that gradually stimulated weak hooves without compromising the horse's comfort.

A similar methodology was developed by K.C. La Pierre, who also advocated a non-invasive trim as a basis for unshod performance.

In parallel with natural hoof care practitioners, these principles were also being used in the Natural Balance shoeing techniques developed by Gene Ovnicek and others.

Sympathetic trimming

Safe, effective trimming is now much more common than it was, and today most good practitioners, whatever their background or training, have a similar, non-invasive approach to their trimming. They will invariably trim in a way which always aims to leave a horse as, or more comfortable after the trim, than he was before.

The most important thing that any hoof care practitioner can do is to listen to the horse. It is never possible to prescribe rules for trimming hooves, since the trim should be as individual as the hoof.

As a result, the hoof care practitioner will need to adapt the way he or she trims to take into account the horse's conformation, the health of the hoof, and the way the horse loads his hoof. Feedback from the horse and the owner are essential, so that the hoof care practitioner can assess whether each trim has improved the horse's way of going or not.

A good hoof care practitioner, no matter how experienced, will normally want to see the horse move before and after he is trimmed, certainly on the first few visits, and regularly after that. They will also question the owner about the way the horse has been performing over a variety of surfaces, if these cannot be seen where the horse is trimmed.

As a general principle, any trim which leaves a horse less sound after the trim than it was before, is a mistake. There may be occasional exceptions, but it should be an extremely rare occurrence for a horse to be less capable after a trim. It is never productive, let alone fair, to make a horse sore, and certainly no horse should be routinely uncomfortable after being trimmed (or shod).

We know that horses' feet are at their healthiest when they are moving a considerable distance each day. We also know that weak hooves respond to appropriate stimulus by growing stronger. It makes sense to ensure that horses are as comfortable as possible, because only by ensuring their comfort can we ensure maximum movement, and only with maximum movement can they grow the healthiest hooves.

With a healthy, barefoot horse, a trim should be a regular part of the horse's routine, but each trim should happen regularly enough that it will only make minor changes to the horse's way of going. Bear in mind that, for the horse, the ideal is for their hooves to be living and working on challenging surfaces, so that they receive plenty of natural wear and stimulus.

Effective trimming should, if possible, mimic this, and not make sudden or severe changes to biomechanics: a good trim should, if anything, enhance the horse's performance.

We will often trim our own horse's hooves the night before a competition, or a day's hunting, so that their feet are at their best.

The hoof care practitioner

The hoof care practitioner has two key responsibilities.

- He or she should be able to give up-to-date advice on the most suitable diet, environment and exercise for the horse.

- He or she should also perform a safe and effective trim on the horse.

Like the other aspects of your horse's hoof care, the trim should be explained to the owner, and the owner should be made aware of the strengths and weaknesses of the horse's hooves, and how they are likely to progress.

Trimming and rehabilitating hooves

Of course, if a horse has weak, compromised hooves, then he will not be as sound or as comfortable as a horse with strong, healthy hooves.

Trimming a horse with weak hooves can feel a bit like walking a tightrope: you need to help bring weak structures back into function, because it is only with stimulus and work that they will strengthen. At the same time, if you over-stress the weak areas, you risk making the horse less, not more, likely to move correctly.

For a horse coming out of shoes, or being rehabilitated from long-term lameness, the hoof care practitioner should agree a programme of trimming, diet and exercise with the horse owner which will optimise the horse's chances of success.

It will be the owner's responsibility to implement any changes which are necessary to the horse's diet, management or exercise regime, but the hoof care practitioner should be able to give detailed advice on these aspects every step of the way.

Rehabilitating a compromised hoof is a form of physiotherapy and, when weak structures are first brought back into work, they will be unable to work hard and will need gradual stimulus in order to improve.

A good example would be the horse on page 126, who had a weak digital cushion and frog, and who required time on conformable surfaces in order to develop. It is important to stimulate the frog and back of the foot as much as possible, but a horse like this would not be comfortable on hard, uneven terrain until he had built up much healthier and tougher structures at the back of the foot.

Generally, as horses grow a better hoof capsule they become steadily more comfortable. Very often, once a horse has grown 50 per cent of his new, well-connected hoof growth, he appears virtually as sound as if he had already grown a whole new hoof capsule.

> The golden rules are that any setback in comfort levels following a trim should:
>
> • Be extremely rare, and never occur when trimming a healthy hoof.
>
> • Only result from new stimulus to a weak part of the hoof (for example, engaging a weak frog or digital cushion), not from invasive trimming.
>
> • Be minor and of short duration (i.e. should last no more than a few days).
>
> • Be easily relieved by putting the horse on supportive footing.

As a caveat, if your horse has been peripherally loading his hoof (either in a shoe or where the hoof wall has become over-long) and, because of dietary overload he has developed sole sensitivity, he will appear 'footier' on uneven ground after being trimmed.

This is because reducing the peripheral loading (by lowering the hoof wall or removing the shoe) also engages the sole. This is not primarily a trimming problem but is something that can only be solved with correct management. Continuing to load the hoof peripherally simply covers up the problem and perpetuates poor hoof function.

Practical advice

We hope that every horse owner wants to know more about the health of their horse's hooves, and how to improve them.

Although we believe that the right trim can only improve a hoof by 10 per cent, or less, in the absence of a correct diet and environment, it is certainly true that hooves can be seriously damaged, and horses seriously injured, by inappropriate trimming.

There are books and websites available which give lots of 'how-to' information about trimming, but in our opinion there is no substitute for hands-on practical training and years of experience.

As a result, this book deliberately does not include specific advice on trimming the hoof, and it is not intended to be a trimming manual.

What we hope is that by looking at trimming as simply one piece in the jigsaw of the horse's hoof, you can put this piece into proportion and take more control over making barefoot work for your horse.

Every hoof and every horse is different, but there are some key guidelines that we believe every hoof care practitioner should follow:

- Listen to the horse: if a trim results in a previously sound horse being less capable, then something is wrong. It is possible to lame a horse with a few poorly-judged strokes of a rasp. If the horse is telling you one thing, but the 'expert' is telling you another, the horse is right and the 'expert' is wrong.

- 'Sometimes, but not always': a trimming technique that is appropriate for one horse will not necessarily be appropriate for another, or even on another hoof on the same horse, particularly where hooves are in need of rehabilitation.

- Most hard-working barefoot horses will grow a new hoof capsule in four to six months. If the horse is not improving over this sort of time period, then re-assess what you and your hoof care professional are doing.

- Look beyond the hoof: the horse's conformation, or old injuries, can have a radical effect on the hoof capsule. Similarly, a horse with apparently poor hoof balance may have pain or weakness in other areas of the body, and this may be affecting how the horse loads his hooves.

- Few horses wear their hooves completely symmetrically, although loading the hoof centrally (rather than peripherally) will encourage symmetry. Uneven wear does not mean that the horse will wear his feet away. In fact, the extra stimulus means that the areas which load more will also grow more and become stronger.

- Remember that trimming is only the 'tip of the iceberg': 10 per cent of building a healthy foot. The horse world, and particularly the barefoot world, tends to be overly obsessed by trimming, given that it makes such a relatively small contribution to a healthy hoof. Remember that it is fundamental to get the horse's diet and environment right (the 90 per cent), before a trim can be truly effective in achieving the final 10 per cent. The responsibility for 90 per cent of a horse's hoof health is therefore in the owner's hands.

Legislation and training for trimming

The training and legal information in this section is correct as at the date of publication, but legislation and regulation can change. For up-to-date information on training and qualifications, you should contact the named organisations directly.

Who can trim?

Under current UK legislation it is legal for anyone to trim a horse's hooves, regardless of whether or not they have adequate training and experience. The only exception is where a hoof is being prepared for shoeing, or having a shoe applied, which, in the UK, can only be carried out by a registered farrier.

There are proposals to introduce voluntary codes of conduct, which are likely to recommend that only qualified hoof care practitioners or farriers should trim professionally. National Occupational standards are now being developed to provide effective, practical training backed up with suitably stringent nationally recognised qualifications. UKNHCP is one of the consultant bodies in this process.

There are no plans, so far as we are aware, for legislation that would restrict trimming by owners on their own horses.

Finding a hoof care professional

There are many different trimming 'schools' in the UK, each with a different philosophy and approach. At the time of writing there is no nationally recognised qualification or standard for trimming, as opposed to farriery, in the UK.

If you are looking for a hoof care professional, word of mouth is often the best way to find someone. Good practitioners will rarely have space on their books, but it may be worth asking to go onto their waiting list or for a recommendation from them to another professional.

The fact that someone is an excellent farrier does not necessarily mean they have experience of barefoot performance horses. Farriers are trained to be specialists in shoeing, not in creating barefoot performance horses, which is a very different discipline. However, there are an increasing number of farriers who have experience of natural hoof care, so it's always worth talking to your farrier first.

Training

There are also several organisations who run training in hoof care in the UK. The UKNHCP, for example, runs courses for professional hoof care practitioners and farriers. Our practitioners are trained specifically in natural hoof care, and unless they are also farriers, will not be qualified to shoe horses.

Some organisations and individuals run short-format, weekend courses aimed at horse owners. While some of these are a valuable way for owners to learn more about their horse's hooves, some purport to teach owners how to trim their own horses over a weekend.

We personally feel that there is more to hoof care than can be learned in a weekend, and that it is often more beneficial for the horse when hoof care is provided by a professional who has had experience of many different horses and hooves.

Details of the main training organisations that run all or part of their training within the UK are set out below, and they will typically have websites that list their qualified practitioners.

Hoof care organisations

UK Natural Hoof Care Practitioners (UKNHCP)

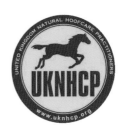

We have to declare our interest here, as we are the founder members of UKNHCP.

This organisation was set up in 2005 to provide training, research and advice to natural hoof care professionals. Members are either farriers who have also trained in natural hoof care or non-farriers who have completed the UKNHCP's training programme.

The programme is specifically designed to give professional hoof care practitioners all the skills they need to improve hoof health and performance in the barefoot horse. It is a modular programme, which takes around eighteen months to complete.

The curriculum is highly practical, and includes anatomy and dissection, equine nutrition, trimming and tool handling, equine behaviour, conformation, rehabilitation and gait analysis, and mentorships with both UK-based and international instructors.

UKNHCP practitioners are required to undertake CPD (continuing professional development) annually to maintain their qualification.

Registered farriers are eligible to train on a shortened course with UKNHCP, and all UKNHCP courses also qualify for CPD points under the Worshipful Company of Farriers' voluntary scheme.

Both students and qualified practitioners are bound by a code of professional conduct, and qualified practitioners carry full professional indemnity insurance. The code of conduct, complaints procedure and the status of practitioners can be checked on the UKNHCP website: www.uknhcp.org

UKNHCP is working with LANTRA (the UK government training body for land-based industries), and with other hoof care organisations, to develop a nationally recognised qualification for natural hoof care which should become a benchmark for future training.

Worshipful Company of Farriers and Farriers' Registration Council

The UK farriery qualification is a four-year course which leads to an NVQ Level 3. This is a detailed course, consisting of theoretical and practical elements, which includes trimming. The emphasis is on making and fitting shoes.

More information can be found at www.farrier-reg.gov.uk

Equine Podiatry (EP)

The term 'equine podiatry' was coined by K.C. La Pierre, an American farrier who runs courses in both the UK and USA.

Equine podiatrists are trained by K.C. La Pierre and are required to undergo both online study and at least twenty-five days practical training.

The course focuses on K.C. La Pierre's own style of trimming, which uses internal and external landmarks to create a 'high-performance trim'.

At the moment, there are two schools of equine podiatry, one based in the UK and one in the US. More information can be found at www.epauk. org (UK) and www.equinepodiatry.net (international).

Association for the Advancement of Natural Horse Care Practices (AANHCP)

This is an American organisation which was founded by Jaime Jackson, and it was one of the original barefoot training organisations. It provides training, in a modular form, most of which is carried out in the US, although some elements can be taken in the UK. Practitioners use the 'wild hoof model' to determine how to trim.

More information is available at www.aanhcp.net

11

Troubleshooting – hoof problems, and how to avoid them

This chapter is a quick-reference guide, and cannot replace advice from a hoof care practitioner and vet: they are the ones who know your horse!

We have listed some of the common hoof problems, with possible causes and preventive measures. Have a look at Chapters 7 and 8 (on diet and environment) as well, which contain lots of practical advice on solving related problems.

While we hope it is helpful, owners should use this chapter with caution – *any severe or prolonged lameness is beyond the scope of this book and should mean an immediate call to your vet!*

Abscesses

Abscesses are much more common in both shod and barefoot horses during periods of prolonged wet weather, when hooves come under persistent attack from bacterial infection.

The onset can be very sudden, with the horse becoming severely lame and unwilling to load the hoof, particularly at the back. However, the horse may have been mildly lame on and off for some time before the abscess causes acute pain.

Solutions and preventative measures

During wet weather, try to allow horses some time each day on dry ground. Ideally, ensure the hoof is as healthy as possible, so that the horse does not have a stretched white line or damaged laminae. A well-connected hoof wall is less prone to infection, and a hard-working hoof with good circulation will fight off infection more quickly.

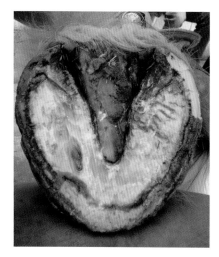

An abscess following a puncture injury to the sole.

Generally, in a healthy hoof, the circulation is sufficiently good that the abscess will resolve fairly quickly, over a few days.

In our experience, barefoot horses will normally blow out abscesses at the coronet or at the top of the heel bulbs, in other words the areas of soft tissue at the top of the hoof capsule.

As a result, trying to relieve an abscess by digging at the sole is rarely totally effective, and can risk opening up routes for further bacterial infection. However, an exception to this might be where a crack is obviously the route of the infection.

The accompanying photo shows a mare who had been barefoot for some years. She had suffered a puncture injury to her sole and developed an abscess some time later. Her vet had tried to relieve the abscess from the sole, but she remained lame and after a couple more days the abscess blew at the coronet, which resolved the lameness.

Bruising

Bruising can occur in a healthy hoof simply as a result of impact while working on hard, stony ground. Bruises of this type appear as small, irregular marks in the wall, often of the hind feet.

Bruising which appears as a horizontal line around the dorsal wall is more serious, and can be a sign of laminitis or bad reaction to a toxin such as a combination wormer. By the time this type of bruising appears, it will unfortunately be too late to prevent the damage.

Bruising in the sole is rare in a healthy hoof, but can occasionally occur. By the time bruising appears in the sole it is normally historic, and not causing the horse an ongoing problem.

A minor bruise on the hoof wall This hoof has just successfully completed a 50-mile endurance race ride.

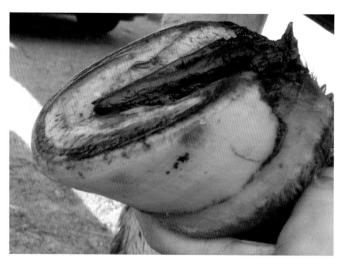

Solutions and preventative measures

Don't worry about bruises in the dorsal wall which simply result from work on challenging surfaces, as these are unlikely to cause the horse any problems.

Of course, if a horse is showing early signs of laminitis then a call to the vet is required, and any ongoing exposure to the potential cause must be removed. For example, if bruising appears after the horse has been turned out on rich pasture, then move the horse and provide safer forage.

Chipping

Hoof wall tends to chip for three main reasons:

1. It may be too long and may have grown proud of the sole.

2. The hoof wall may be of poor quality, flared or separated.

3. The hoof wall may have been weakened, above the chipping, by nail holes, which allow fungal invasion of the hoof wall.

Solutions and preventative measures

Nail holes Time and hoof growth will take care of this. There should only be very slight chipping provided the hooves are trimmed regularly, and better hoof growth should mean the old nail holes grow out within six to eight weeks.

Long wall Hoof wall, a few millimetres of keratin, is not strong enough to bear the weight of the horse on its own, if it has grown longer than other structures of the hoof. Hoof wall that is too long will naturally chip; this can be solved by more frequent trimming.

Poor or flared hoof wall

Most commonly, in our experience, poor quality hoof wall is a result of a dietary imbalance or mineral deficiency, coupled with a lack of stimulus. This type of hoof wall is brittle, and often occurs in conjunction with stretch in the white line. In both cases, the integrity of the connection between the hoof wall and internal structures is inadequate, resulting in the hoof wall chipping. Resolve the dietary or mineral problem, increase the stimulus to the hoof wall, and chipping will also cease to be a problem.

Contracted heels

Contracted heels occur more frequently in shod horses, but are not solely a shoeing problem, and it is equally possible for unshod horses to suffer from contracted heels.

There are two main contributory factors: high heels, and lack of engagement of the back of the foot. Once a horse has a high heel, the frog becomes less actively engaged, and eventually if this is perpetuated, the heels will contract. Once the heels start to contract, the frog becomes even less engaged and will be prone to central sulcus infections, thrush or even canker.

Solutions and preventative measures

A horse with contracted heels has a weak back of the foot, and needs a more holistic approach than simply lowering the heels or shortening the toe.

Both of these trimming processes will need to occur at some point, but since this type of trim will force the horse to engage the back of the foot, it must be done slowly and sympathetically, in conjunction with an environment and exercise programme which will strengthen the back of the foot. Lower heels may also affect muscles, tendons and ligaments above. This should be taken into account before any action is taken.
Heels will de-contract fairly quickly, given the opportunity, but it takes longer to rebuild the digital cushion and lateral cartilages.

The accompanying photos show the same hoof on the day it was de-shod and then two months later. The frog in this type of hoof is often susceptible to thrush so until it is totally healthy, it may be beneficial to use an antiseptic solution to prevent bacterial and fungal infection. Your hoof care practitioner will be able to advise on effective topical treatments.

Contracted heels before (LEFT) and after (RIGHT) treatment.

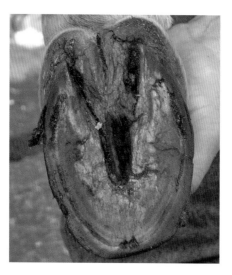 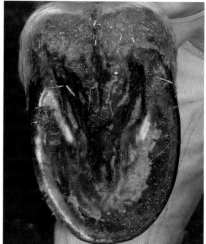

Cracks

Cracks have a variety of causes, and all cracks will worsen if they are subjected to force.

Cracks which begin from the coronet are commonly the result of either damage to the coronet, which has caused a permanent defect in the hoof wall produced at that point, or mechanical forces on the hoof. The mechanical forces may (rarely) arise from imbalanced loading; or be a consequence of structural weakness at the back of the hoof.

Much more common are cracks which are worse at ground level, and which result from pressure on weak or over-long hoof wall. Quarter cracks are a classic example.

Toe cracks can also fall into this category, but can also be caused by a defect in the sole at the toe, which leads to a lack of attachment in the hoof wall at this point. As breakover puts considerable pressure on the hoof wall at the toe, a toe crack is likely to result at the location of the defect.

Solutions and preventative measures

Correct trimming is essential to relieve or minimise the forces on cracks. This will improve all cracks, but will not necessarily resolve them fully.

Our experience is that cracks heal well in barefoot horses. The trim needs to relieve mechanical forces. Correct biomechanical movement needs to strengthen the back of the hoof and additional stimulus to the hoof wall allows it to thicken, stabilising cracks from within.

Any areas of fungal infection will need to be treated at the same time, since fungal infection can perpetuate cracks.

Often there will be a cavity behind the crack which fills with debris; this can perpetuate or make the crack worse. Regularly cleaning the debris out of the cavity, treating it with an antibacterial and fungal solution and then plugging it with cotton wool, will ensure it stays clean while it is healing.

Flat feet

In our opinion flat feet are rarely a function of genetics alone. We have seen many flat feet build concavity once diet and environment have improved. Typically, flat feet which are the result of dietary problems also have poor quality hoof wall and may have a stretched white line.

Don't confuse lack of concavity with flat feet, however. Concavity is dictated by the environment the horses lives and works in, and deeper concavity is not necessarily better (see page 30).

Solutions and preventative measures

The best remedy for flat feet is time, coupled with a correct diet, which will allow a better-connected hoof capsule to grow. The plaster casts on page 70 show clearly how concavity builds once the entire hoof capsule has a strong connection between the hoof wall and internal structures, the result of a healthy laminar connection.

Weak or crumbly hoof wall

This is normally a result of poor diet, mineral deficiencies or simply lack of stimulus.

Solutions and preventative measures

By implementing changes to diet and environment, and increasing stimulus to the hoof in a way which keeps the horse comfortable, it is possible to rapidly improve hoof wall quality, as the photos on page 15 demonstrate.

Stretched white line/'seedy toe'/'white line disease'

A stretched white line results from inflammation and damage to the laminae, which causes the bond between the hoof wall and the sensitive internal structures to weaken.

All horses with clinical laminitis will have a stretched white line. This can also occur in horses who have not developed full-blown laminitis but may be showing mild, sub-clinical signs, like sole sensitivity.

Once a stretched white line has developed, the horse will be at greater risk of suffering from abscesses. The holes created by the stretch can be an easy route via which infection can attack the hoof. It is also possible for tiny stones to lodge in these holes, but contrary to popular belief, these are an effect of the stretched white line, not a cause. It is simply not possible for stones to penetrate a healthy white line, because with healthy laminae, the hoof wall is so tightly bonded to the internal structures that there are no holes.

Ironically, 'seedy toe' and 'white line disease' will only occur where the white line is already seriously compromised.

Solutions and preventative measures

A stretched white line is always indicative of a poor diet, mineral deficiencies, or a toxin which is affecting the metabolism. These toxins can be as the result of external ingestion (as with wormers) or they may be produced in the horse's body as a result of an illness.

Once the white line has stretched, it cannot heal – the only way to resolve the problem is for a better connected hoof capsule to grow down.

If the cause is a poor diet or mineral deficiencies, these can be resolved fairly easily, and the dietary advice in Chapter 7 is a good starting point.

If the hoof does not respond to dietary improvements, then it becomes more likely that the horse's metabolism has been compromised. Veterinary advice is essential here; insulin resistance and exposure to toxins are common causes of damage to the horse's metabolism, and a detailed diagnosis and treatment programme will be required, in addition to effective hoof care.

Thin soles

It is rare for a healthy barefoot horse to have a thin sole, as in a healthy, hardworking hoof the sole builds thickness and depth in response to stimulus. However, in horses who have a metabolic illness the hoof may flare and the sole stretch with the increasing girth of the hoof.

The sole of a barefoot horse should not be trimmed, as this structure provides essential protection when horses are working on challenging surfaces.

Thin soles are a fairly common problem for some horses in shoes and can be caused either by trimming, or by lack of stimulus.

Occasionally, a previously healthy horse will develop a soft sole, most evident round the apex of the frog. We have observed that this occurs in horses in localised areas, and with some horses, but not all, it is improved when they are given additional dietary zinc. Not all horses improve, though, so this is far from conclusive.

Solutions and preventative measures

Thin soles are very vulnerable, and it is particularly important that they are protected if a horse has metabolic issues or when coming out of shoes.

Conformable surfaces allow the sole to be supported while it receives the stimulus needed to thicken and develop. Hoof boots can be a useful measure to protect the sole if working the horse on hard ground is unavoidable.

Thrush or fungal infection

In mild, damp climates, fungal infection and thrush are common problems, seizing any opportunity to attack weak hooves, and particularly weak frogs.

Once established, fungal infection can be very persistent, attacking the central sulcus of the frog, in particular.

Solutions and preventative measures

Getting rid of fungal infection involves a two-pronged approach. A topical anti-fungal treatment is the starting point, but this will only keep the infection at bay.

The second essential is to improve the overall hoof health. Fungal infection can lead to a vicious circle where, because of a tender, infected frog, the horse does not engage the back of his hoof. Lacking stimulus, the frog then weakens, and becomes even more prone to infection.

By contrast, a healthy frog will have no weak spots or pockets where infection can lurk, and so will fight off fungal infection in wet conditions. Even in the wettest climate, healthy frogs attached to healthy hooves will not succumb to fungal infection, and will never need topical treatments.

Providing stimulating, well-drained surfaces for the horse to live and work on helps the frog become stronger and healthier. The wetter the climate, the more imperative it is to give the hooves regular time on dry ground.

Providing the correct diet will also allow the hoof capsule to suspend the frog correctly. A squashed frog under a collapsed hoof capsule will be weaker and susceptible to opportunist bugs and thus infection.

Toe-dubbing

Toe-dubbing is the name we use to describe the wear that some horses show in the dorsal wall, above the normal point of breakover. This normally occurs in hind feet, and can be bilateral or unilateral.

Horses who toe-dub, instead of simply wearing the hoof wall at ground level, in normal breakover, wear the dorsal hoof wall as well when the hoof drags on the ground at the toe. In severe cases, the outer dorsal wall can be worn away back to the white line in that area.

This is always a mechanical problem, caused either by lack of flexibility in a joint in the affected limb, or by an excessively long toe (perhaps owing to laminitis or a long under-run hoof).

Solutions and preventative measures

If the toe-dubbing is a result of a long, under-run hoof then, as the overall health and function of the hoof improves, the toe-dubbing will disappear. Similarly, if it is a result of laminitis, then it will resolve itself once a better-connected hoof wall has grown down.

Long-term toe-dubbing in an otherwise healthy hoof is often an indication of reduced joint flexibility, commonly in the hock, stifle or sacro-iliac. The vet, possibly working with an equine bodyworker, such as a physiotherapist, needs to advise on the best solution, and once full joint flexion has been re-established, the toe-dubbing will cease.

In some horses, it may not be possible to restore joint flexion completely. It is worth noting that, even though toe-dubbing leads to excessive wear of the dorsal hoof wall, it rarely seems to cause a problem in the hoof itself.

12

Why barefoot – what next?

Science is now beginning to allow the horse to tell his own story…at this late date in the history of man and horse, it is only the objective tools of science that can sort out what millenniums of tradition, lore and wishful thinking have sometimes muddled.

Stephen Budiansky, *The Nature of Horses*, 1997.

We have proved that many different breeds of horse in the UK can work hard in every discipline without shoes.

Today, we have horses with healthy hooves: their hooves meet our benchmark by being capable of going over challenging surfaces at any gait, day after day.

However, there was a time when we were unaware of the choice we as owners could make. In addition, until we gave our horses the right diet, environment and exercise their hooves were neither as healthy nor as capable as they are today.

As the years have gone by, we have found that there are also huge benefits to working horses without shoes.

Horses without shoes injure themselves less, and do less damage with their feet than shod horses – whether this is while they are in motion, travelling in a trailer or horsebox, when they tread on your toes or when they kick out at another horse.

Research in humans has shown that runners with bare feet absorb shock better, have greater proprioception, and suffer fewer injuries, than those who wear shoes. Our experience of riding horses on varied terrain suggests that this is also true of barefoot horses.

There is the added advantage of never having to cancel a competition or cut short a day's riding because of lost shoes.

Riders of barefoot horses often comment that they feel less concussion than when their horses were shod. Barefoot horses seem to have superior ability to adapt to impact forces, with their hooves giving a cushioned ride. One rider said that, when riding his newly barefoot mare, it felt as if she had air suspension trainers, instead of the hob-nailed boots of when she was shod.

It is certainly true that a bare hoof with a strong digital cushion, healthy lateral cartilages and a well-developed vascular system has incredible shock-absorbing properties, and that these same properties are less developed when the back of the foot is restricted by a shoe.

Now that natural hoof care is becoming more popular, and more owners are interested in working their horses without shoes, there should be more opportunities for research into healthy hoof function and how this is achieved or lost.

You can see that all parts of healthy hooves have a function – they do not require all the horse's weight to be loaded onto the periphery of the hoof.

We now question whether peripherally loading the hoof, nailing steel or gluing plastic onto a biological structure, could ever be as effective as allowing the hoof to develop its full range of natural function. We now question the traditional thinking that says that shoes applied to the hoof make it stronger.

Dogs, cats, humans, sheep, cattle, deer – in fact every animal you can think of – all load the whole foot, not just the periphery.

Are horses so different? By treating them differently are we helping or harming them?

13

Case studies

Lucy

History

Long-term laminitis, shod in regular shoes but often lame or pottery.

Diet from the day the shoes were removed

Ad lib late-cut hay, turnout in totally grass-free area 20 x 20 m (66 x 66 ft) half concrete/half wood bark. (See photo and related text on page 109.) Small feed of unmolassed beet pulp given twice daily to give supplements of seaweed, linseed, brewers' yeast, magnesium and *agnus castus* (see Glossary).

Existing exercise

Turned out 24 hours during summer, periods of box rest when laminitic, then restricted grazing on a starvation patch. Stabled at night, and out during the day during winter. Driven and ridden when soundness allowed.

Exercise programme over rehabilitation period

1 year: Daily exercise in padded boots, driving or ridden, which is at least an hour's exercise at walk unless Lucy wants to go faster! Lucy not able to tolerate hard or stony surfaces without boots on in front, but happy to have bare hind feet. She seems to have good periods and bad periods with no clear reason why.

18 months: A blood test reveals severe insulin resistance, daily dose of Metformin prescribed.

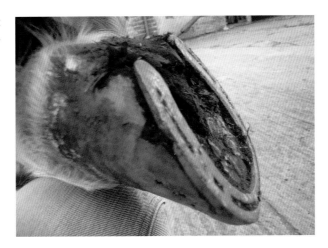

Lucy's left forefoot at the start of treatment.

20 months: Lucy's environment changed to a very large area of concrete buildings and tracks around which she can wander 24 hours a day with a companion horse. Hay is placed around this environment to make Lucy move, thus increasing the level of exercise she receives. All previous diet and exercise in boots continues.

2 years: All previous exercise in boots continues but now Lucy is also happy to pull her cart unbooted along smooth tarmac surfaces. Her hoof sensitivity has dramatically decreased the more she has roamed her large track and concrete environment.

2½ years: Lucy put back into her original 20 x 20 m (66 x 66 ft) environment to avoid summer grass growing around the edges of the tracks in the other environment. She is now not on Metformin or *agnus castus* but is the best she has ever been. She is exercised every day either in her cart or by racing around a small field. She seems to know this is just for exercise and is quite happy in her grass-free home with ad lib hay.

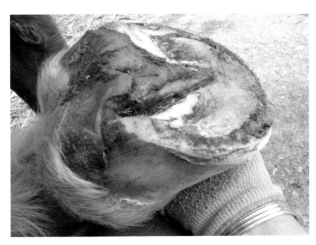

Lucy's left forefoot after nearly three years of treatment.

3 years: Lucy continues to make extraordinary progress. Her hooves, although still very compromised, show less white line stretch at the toe and she is happy on all but the most challenging of surfaces. Her owners continue to boot her in front unless they are working purely on soft or smooth surfaces. She no longer requires pads in her boots.

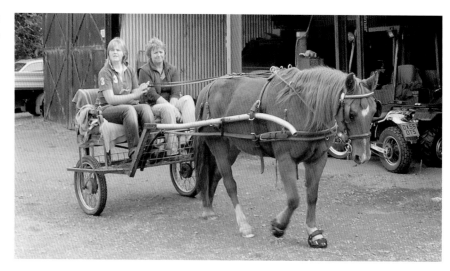

Lucy being driven on a road surface.

After following the diet and exercise advice to the letter, Lucy started to improve very slowly, but we knew it would be a slow, long process. Her hooves and her health were in a very bad state. She was on a strictly no grass or titbits diet; only hay, Speedibeet and her minerals. We gradually built up her exercise regime and noticed that the more exercise she had, the more she improved. Three years down the line we've got the old Lucy back, giving the family so much fun and enjoyment.

SUE AND RACHEL VERNON

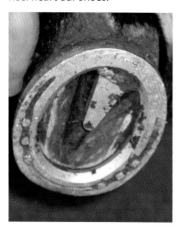

Foxy shod with raised heel heart bar shoes.

Foxy

History

Lame left fore and, after investigation, diagnosed with navicular. Shod with raised heel heart bars, in which he was sound, albeit with a very short, choppy stride, when removed in May.

Diet from the day the shoes were removed

Ad lib late-cut meadow-grass haylage, virtually grass-free on a track system.

One daily feed consisting of:

1 kg (2 lb 3 oz) alfalfa
1 kg (2 lb 3 oz) unmolassed sugar beet
100 g (3½ oz) seaweed
50 g (1¼ oz) brewer's yeast
50 g (1¼ oz) magnesium
250 g (9 oz) micronised linseed
1 kg (2 lb 3 oz) copra meal – reduced to 0.5 kg (1 lb 2 oz) at 12 weeks

Existing exercise

Stabled with no turnout for previous seven months; ridden under saddle in an arena and on the beach. Short periods of lungeing, although this was difficult because of behavioural problems.

Exercise programme over rehabilitation period

6 weeks: On a track with varied surfaces – pea gravel, road planings, earth, limestone hardcore with crushed surface. Led out in walk, from another horse, along roads with some trotting if soundness allowed, twice a week. Work in hand, establishing groundwork in an arena and field, no limit.

7–8 weeks: Ridden work at walk and trot in arena and field, straight lines, no circles, no limit. Hacking to an arena in walk along roads, round trip of 9.5 km (6 miles), once per week. Other hacking for an hour twice per week amounting to roads and soft surfaces in walk and trot.

9–10 weeks: Ridden work at walk, trot and canter in field, introducing jumps. Hacking to an arena in walk and trot along roads, round trip of 9.5 km (6 miles), once per week. Other hacking for an hour twice per week on roads and soft surfaces in walk, trot and canter. At the end of this period Foxy attended a local Riding Club show-jumping clinic.

11–12 weeks: All previous exercise continues. Trip to show-jumping competition and local 9.5-km (6-mile) all grass cross-country course. At the end of week 12 Foxy completed a 10-mile fun ride on a variety of terrain.

13–14 weeks: All previous exercise continues. Show-jumping competition and four and half hours hunting with the Exmoor Foxhounds.

15–16 weeks: Lame right fore and very reluctant to land heel-first, pointing foot when standing. No exercise apart from turnout while lame. Over the next ten days lameness improves and then he is sound at all gaits on the soft but reluctant to stride out downhill on roads. Exercise resumed once sound.

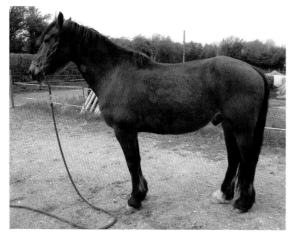
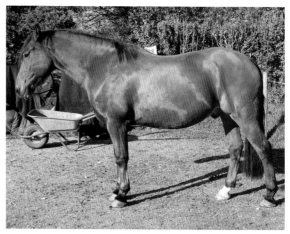

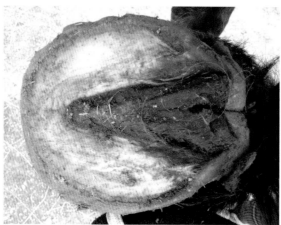
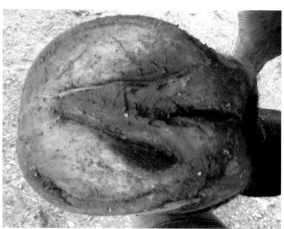

TOP LEFT AND RIGHT These two photos show how Foxy developed physically over a five-month period.

BELOW LEFT AND RIGHT Changes to Foxy's right forefoot during the same period.

17 weeks: 10-mile fun ride with jumps on predominantly soft terrain, clear round and novice show-jumping competition.

18 weeks: Lameness in right fore returns accompanied by pus exuding from central sulcus. Soak hoof in a poultice boot in a salt water solution twice per day. Three days later the heel bulbs split and this creates an exit for the infection. Foxy is sound intermittently but unhappy when travelling over rough terrain.

19 weeks: Deep central sulcus infection still evident when hoof pick inserted into the central sulcus of the hoof on the right fore. Start to flush the crack with salt water through a syringe and then fill with Manuka honey and pack with cotton wool soaked in antibiotic solution. By the end of the week the sulcus is opening up and looking clean. Foxy is now happy along all the road planing tracks.

20 weeks: Exercise resumed to previous level, plus 10-mile fun ride with jumps over varied terrain.

21 weeks: Novice level hunter trial completed in great style, plus flatwork and hacking.

22 weeks: 10-mile fun ride with jumps, plus flatwork and hacking.

23 weeks: 10-mile fun ride with jumps, plus flatwork and hacking.

24 weeks: 10-mile fun ride with jumps, plus flatwork and hacking.

25 weeks: Drag hunting for four hours, novice show-jumping, plus flatwork and hacking.

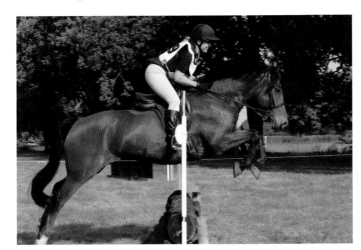

Foxy competing successfully in a hunter trial.

Devon

History

Ten years old. Sound in shoes, no known problems although owner was concerned that his heels had become increasingly under-run over the years that Devon had been shod.

Diet started 4 weeks before the shoes were removed

Diet changed in mid-February, shoes off mid-March.
Daily feed (soaked in one and half buckets of water) consisting of:

3 kg (6 lb 9 oz) lucerne nuts
1 kg (2 lb 3 oz) unmolassed dried
    sugar-beet pulp
1 kg (2 lb 3 oz) lucerne chop
400 g (14 oz) linseed meal
seaweed

brewers' yeast
cider vinegar
magnesium powder
rock-salt lick in stable
Ad lib hay/haylage

Existing exercise

Out during day, stabled at night. Ridden at a variety of Riding Club events, dressage to Medium level. Ridden six days per week.

Exercise programme over rehabilitation period

4 weeks: Daily exercise on soft surfaces in all gaits. Short periods in hand in walk on tarmac, no longer than half an hour. Time to be reduced if Devon appears short-striding, but most days he is taken for short walks in hand up the road after exercise. Two days after his shoes come off Devon competes at Riding Club show-jumping with no ill-effects. He does slip on a muddy corner at a hunter trial but this is only a week after his shoes came off.

5–8 weeks: All previous exercise but lengthened hacks in walk, trot and canter on soft or conformable surfaces only. Devon has normally worn boots for his forefeet but only needs them a couple of times on hacks where there are more stones. Smooth tarmac is no problem but the gravel on the road is a little difficult.

9–12 weeks: All previous exercise, but now including short periods of trot work on the road whenever Devon is forward-going. He is now able to canter along verges, and gravel is becoming less of a problem. He does not wear boots at all in this period, which includes a 10-mile fun ride with lots of jumps and canters over mixed terrain.

13–16 weeks: All previous exercise plus Devon competes in a Riding Club one-day event qualifier with no slippage in any phase, although his owner rides cautiously on the cross-country course.

17–20 weeks: All previous exercise plus attendance at a Riding Club camp where Devon does show-jumping and cross-country on grass with more confidence. Dressage on the all-weather surface is never a problem and quite

BELOW LEFT Devon's left forefoot seen shod in March.

BELOW RIGHT The same forefoot unshod in September.

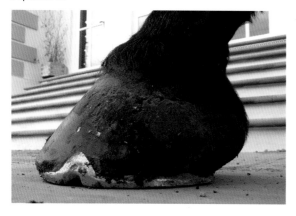
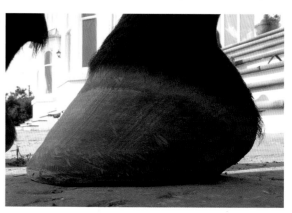

spectacular at times. During this period he also does Riding Club dressage qualifiers at Elementary and Medium levels on grass with no caution and no slip-ups, and is placed in both classes.

6–8 months: Devon does a Riding Club show-jumping qualifier on grass, and for the first time Devon's owner rides without thinking about having no shoes or studs. No problems and is placed in both classes. Hacks out without problems for up to an hour and a half.

(During his seventh month going barefoot, the day before a one-day event Devon was slightly lame on the near fore, which has always been his worst foot. On poulticing some 'gunk' came out and a few days later he was sound. This was the only time during the rehabilitation that he was lame. Since then he has had no problems and he is now walking as he did when he was three years old, heel first.)

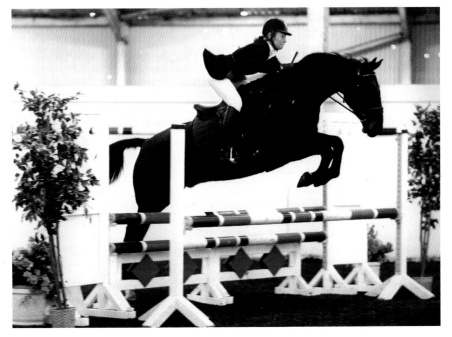

Devon showjumping successfully.

I was pleasantly surprised how simple the transition was and how quickly Devon grew himself a new set of feet. Really interesting to watch the angle of growth change to how it used to be when he was young, which had been what I had been observing go wrong over the past few years. Living in such a hilly area with slippery tarmac everywhere I am so impressed with the new non-slip soles Devon has grown for roadwork and amazed at the capacity of hoof to grow as quickly as I can wear it out on the road. No 'bleeding stumps' so far! In less than a year I have been utterly convinced that there are many reasons for opening our minds to non-traditional ways of managing our horses and have had shattered some of the preconceptions I have had regarding the capacity of my horse's hoof to withstand anything I can throw at it, provided I put in place the things he needs to do his part.

JO ELLIS

Mick

History

Remedial farriery to correct medial cracks in both front hooves for two years. Treatment consisted of opening up the cracks with a dremel, filling with epoxy resin and then pinning horizontally to effect healing. Bar shoes and rim shoes were used. Box rest was prescribed for long periods but after eighteen months the crack on the right fore was bleeding from the coronary band. Further remedial work repeating the epoxy resin and pinning was unsuccessful for four months after the bleeding started. At the time of shoe removal Mick's hooves showed very poor development of the lateral cartilages and digital cushion. The heels on his right fore were showing signs of becoming sheared owing to the weakness in the back third of the hoof.

Diet from the day the shoes were removed

Reduced grass where possible but difficult because of livery arrangements. Havens (German) Slobbermash and Cool Mix with a handful Hi-fi plus 50 grams (about 1¾ oz) of magnesium oxide daily.

Existing exercise

Unable to be exercised because of severe cracks; periods of box rest difficult because of behavioural problems. Crack in right fore would bleed when low-level exercise carried out. It was suggested that Mick should be box-rested for a year.

Exercise programme over rehabilitation period

4 weeks: Daily exercise on soft surfaces at walk only for half an hour. This consists of riding in a field and down some grassy tracks. Mick is also turned out in a small paddock 24 hours per day. He is given hay once the grass has been eaten down. All ridden exercise stops if bleeding occurs at the coronary band in the right fore.

5–8 weeks: All exercise as before, still in walk, but lengthened daily to an hour as no bleeding has occurred from the coronary band.

9–12 weeks: All previous exercise but including periods of walk and trot on the road. Mick and his owner enjoy going to a local cross-country event, but they don't go over the jumps; Mick is also taken to the beach.

1. Mick's right forefoot before the second remedial treatment.

2. Mick's right forefoot after the removal of shoes and a further four months of remedial farriery.

13–22 weeks: Mick has had no lameness or bleeding and the crack is starting to grow out at the coronary band. Exercise at all gaits is now included and some jumping over obstacles no higher than 60 cm (2 ft). Mick is sound on all but the most challenging of surfaces.

23 weeks: Mick attends his first competitive event in two years, a local Riding Club show-jumping competition. He is continuing with all previous exercise and the cracks are healing.

3. Considerable improvement in Mick's right forefoot, but still the stubborn remnants of the condition.

6 months–1 year: Mick can be ridden in all activities as a normal horse and attends a three-day Riding Club camp at Somerford Park in Cheshire, where he takes part in dressage, show-jumping and cross-country lessons in the same way as all the shod horses. He is sound and happy on all but the most challenging of surfaces. This could possibly be improved if he were kept on a different diet, but as his owner rides and hacks on surfaces on which Mick is comfortable, further changes are unnecessary. The cracks continue to heal; they are still visible but are causing no further problems.

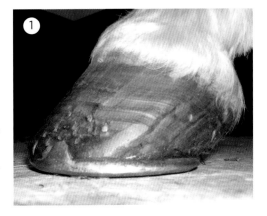

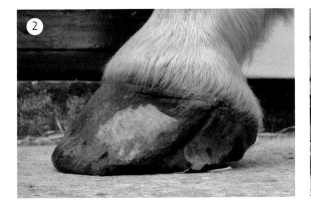

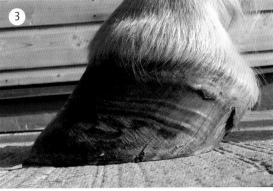

After continual remedial farriery for years, lameness and being advised by vets to box-rest Mick for a year I had nothing to lose by going barefoot. Mick adapted very quickly to being without shoes – in fact it hardly affected him. His feet look the best they've ever been, with the cracks almost grown out, but more importantly they've healed on the inside.

Almost instantly Mick was back in full work, enjoying cross-country, fun rides and hacks. Going barefoot was the best decision for both Mick and myself – it's amazing to see his improvement and to know that he is happy and comfortable now.

LYNDA GARDINER

Mick jumping.

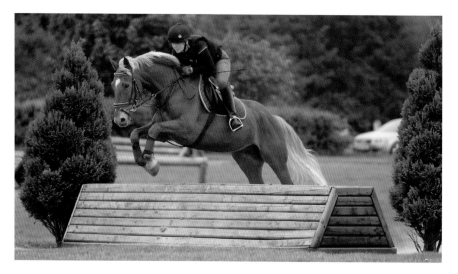

Bill

History

Bill was 12-year-old ID x TB with prolonged lameness in the left fore, high heels and long toes. Diagnosed with navicular but digital radiographs revealed sidebone and ringbone, as well as a weak digital cushion and poor medial/lateral balance. Arrived in shoes with pronounced toe-first landing.

Diet from the day the shoes were removed

Ad lib organic meadow haylage
Grazing at night
Seaweed, brewers' yeast, linseed, calcined magnesite (in quantities consistent with those advised in Table 2 in Chapter 7)
Unmolassed sugar beet, unmolassed alfalfa, copra meal (as had poor topline and muscle atrophy)

Previous management

Stabled at night, out during day. Occasionally lunged, but had not been in work for at least eighteen months prior to rehabilitation.

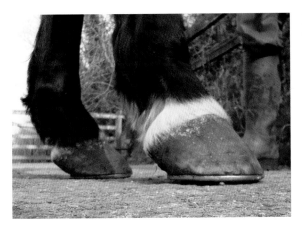
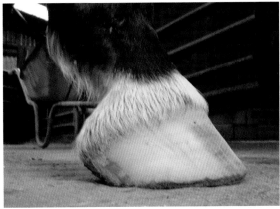

Bill's right forefoot in April (LEFT) and after about five months (RIGHT).

Exercise programme over rehabilitation period

1–15 weeks: No work. Turned out on grass or pea gravel track and yard to ensure comfort levels. Unlevel and landing toe-first on concrete. Uncomfortable on turns.

16–20 weeks: Finally landing heel-first and level, after growing 75 per cent of a new, healthier and better connected hoof capsule. Fantastic improvement in hoof shape. Work starts from scratch, initially led from another horse but quickly progressing to ridden work.

21 weeks onwards: Ridden work on all surfaces, increasing as fitness improves. Six months after entering rehabilitation, this horse is able to start hunting and jumping again.

Bill out hunting after his rehabilitation.

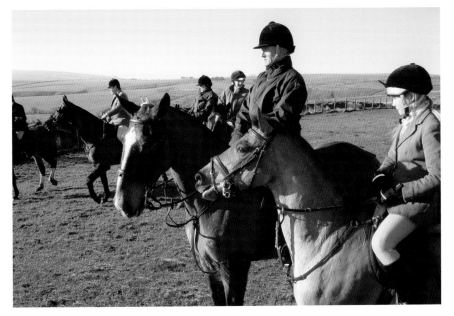

Hector

History

Hector was a six-year-old Irish Sport Horse with bilateral lameness, worse on the left fore. He was short-striding in front, with a weak right hind and severe muscle wastage over the gluteal mass and hamstrings in his right hind. He arrived in shoes with pronounced toe-first landing. Likely that only soft tissue damage was contributing to lameness.

Diet from the day the shoes were removed

Ad lib organic meadow haylage
Grazing at night (through spring and summer only)
Seaweed, brewers' yeast, linseed, calcined magnesite (in quantities consistent with those advised in Table 2 in Chapter 7)
Unmolassed sugar beet, unmolassed alfalfa, copra meal

Previous management

Young event horse, but vet's opinion was that he was unsuitable and had no future because of the lameness.

Exercise programme over rehabilitation period

1–2 weeks: No work. Turned out on grass or pea gravel track and yard to ensure comfort levels.

2–4 weeks: Already landing heel-first and much better on tough surfaces than on arrival. Ridden work commences, over all surfaces, but limited work on rough, stony ground.

Hector's sole in July (BELOW LEFT) and November (BELOW RIGHT).

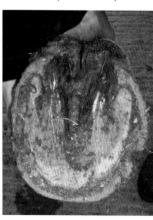
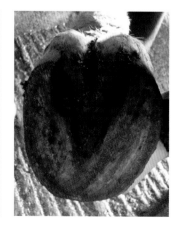

4–8 weeks: Ridden work on all surfaces, increasing as fitness improves. Hector is now capable of at least an hour of road-work daily and his movement is competent on stony ground.

8 weeks onwards: Hector starts hunting, and takes to it like a duck to water! He hunts three times a fortnight from then on, over all terrain. Within five months of his shoes coming off he has grown a complete new hoof capsule, with a better

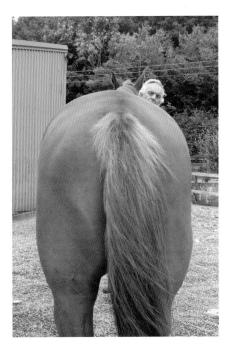 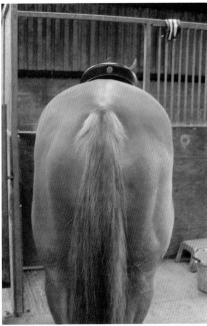

As improvement in his feet allowed more work, Hector's muscle wastage disappeared and his new muscular development was much more even. Compare his gluteal region in July (LEFT) with how he looked by October (RIGHT).

connected hoof wall, shorter toe, and compact, shock-absorbing digital cushion. His muscular development has become much more even now that he is sound on his left fore/right hind, and previous wastage has disappeared.

He moves beautifully, and goes over jumps as athletically as a cat! He's got a new lease of life!

HECTOR'S RIDER

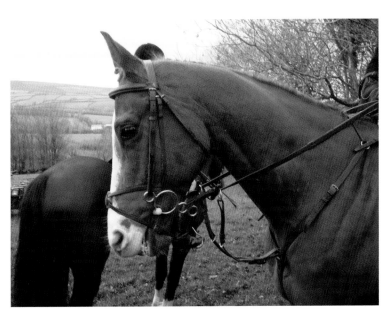

Hector took to hunting like a duck to water.

Posy

History

Posy was a nine-year-old Thoroughbred mare with prolonged lameness to the left fore; thin-soled and very 'footy'. Diagnosed with navicular/deep digital flexor tendonitis on the basis of nerve blocks and radiographs. Remedial shoeing had not led to improvement, and at the start of rehabilitation she had a pronounced toe-first landing. She also had a history of muscle pain in the neck and shoulders, probably a by-product of foot pain.

Diet from the day the shoes were removed

Ad lib organic meadow haylage
Grazing at night (through spring and summer, restricted if she appeared 'footy' on stones)
Seaweed, brewers' yeast, linseed, calcined magnesite (in quantities consistent with those advised in Table 2 in Chapter 7)
Unmolassed sugar beet, unmolassed alfalfa, crushed oats (varied amounts depending on work level)

Previous management

Stabled at night, out during day. Described as 'sharp'. Worked in school and over jumps, occasional hacking.

Exercise programme over rehabilitation period

1–4 weeks: No work. Turned out on grass or pea gravel track and yard to ensure comfort levels. 'Footy' on concrete.

4–6 weeks: Worked in hand and led from another horse on good surfaces only. No roadwork.

6–8 weeks: Comfortable on concrete, started work led from another horse on good surfaces (half hour rising to one hour).

8+ weeks: Ridden work on all surfaces, plus roadwork (up to half hour every other day). Jumping introduced, along with hill work for fitness.

10+ weeks: Started competitions, including hunter trialling. Hacking or hill work daily over varied terrain. Horse now landing confidently heel-first over all surfaces and at all gaits.

Barefoot – Discovery or Delay?

Think for a moment what surgery was like before the invention of anaesthesia in 1842…Imagine taking pride above all in the speed with which you wield the knife…speed was essential, for the shock of an operation could itself be a major factor in bringing about the patient's death.

Now think about this: in 1795 a doctor discovered that inhaling nitrous oxide killed pain…yet no surgeon experimented with this…The use of anaesthetics was pioneered not by surgeons but by humble dentists.

One of the first practitioners of painless dentistry, Horace Wells, was driven to suicide by the hostility of the medical profession.

When anaesthesia was first employed in London in 1846 it was called a 'Yankee dodge'. In other words, practising anaesthesia felt like cheating. Most of the characteristics that the surgeon had developed – the indifference, the strength, the pride, the sheer speed – were suddenly irrelevant.

Why did it take 50 years to invent anaesthesia? Any answer has to recognise the emotional investment surgeons had made in becoming a certain sort of person with a certain sort of skills and the difficulty of abandoning that self-image.

…If we turn to other discoveries, we find that they too have the puzzling feature of unnecessary delay…*if we start looking at progress we find we actually need to tell a story of delay as well as a story of discovery, and in order to make sense of these delays we need to turn away from the inflexible logic of discovery and look at other factors: the role of the emotions, the limits of the imagination, the conservatism of institutions.*

…If you want to think about what progress really means, then you need to imagine what it was like to have become so accustomed to the screams of patients that they seemed perfectly natural and normal…you must first understand what stands in the way of progress.

From *Bad Medicine* by David Wootton, by permission
of Oxford University Press

Glossary

Agnus castus Herbal remedy used as a treatment for horses with insulin resistance or Cushing's syndrome.

Barefoot A domesticated horse who is working without shoes.

Breakover The area of the toe which is the last to leave the ground at the final phase of the stride.

Conformable surface A surface, such as pea gravel or sand, which supports and loads the whole hoof.

Corium (solar or frog) The internal vascularised structure from which the sole/frog is produced.

Dorsal wall The outer aspect of the hoof wall from coronet to toe.

Fructan The main carbohydrate found in UK grasses.

Growth rings Horizontal ridges or ripples in the external hoof wall.

Insulin resistance A metabolic disorder where horses have high levels of blood-glucose and are prone to sudden bouts of laminitis.

Laminae The interlocking tissues which form the junction between the hoof capsule and the internal structures of the hoof.

Laminitis Inflammation of the laminae, resulting in foot pain and loss of attachment of the hoof capsule to the internal structures of the hoof.

Lateral The aspect of the hoof further from the midline of the horse's body.

Medial The aspect of the hoof closer to the midline of the horse's body.

Natural hoof care The practice of keeping horses barefoot, encompassing trimming, nutrition, environmental considerations and exercise.

Navicular syndrome Term used as an umbrella for lameness associated with pain in the palmar aspect of the hoof; now understood to frequently be the result of soft tissue damage rather than primarily navicular bone degeneration.

Palmar The aspect of the hoof closer to the back of the forelimb.

Pea gravel Rounded 5–10 mm (⅕–⅖ in) gravel, a supportive surface for weak hooves.

Perfusion A term used to describe the pressure of blood flow through the capillaries.

Plantar The aspect of the hoof closer to the back of the hind limb.

Peripheral loading Loading the hoof capsule and limb by restricting weight-bearing to the hoof wall, as in a shod hoof.

Proprioception Awareness of the position of the body from neural receptors (in the context of this book, those in the hoof).

Unshod In the context of this book, this term is used to refer to horses who have no shoes on but are not in work (e.g: retired horses, companions, broodmares, youngstock), i.e. as distinct from horses who are working barefoot.

Venous plexus A network of veins and capillaries in the foot.

References

1 Siff and Verkhosansky, *Supertraining* (4th edn), (Denver, Colorado) 1999.

2 Robbins and Hanna, 'Running-related injury prevention through barefoot adaptations', *Medicine and Science in Sports and Exercise* 19, (1987), pp.148–156.

3 Robbins et al, (1990) 'Athletic footwear and chronic overloading: a brief review', *Sports Medicine* 9, (1990), pp.76–85.

4 Robbins et al, 'Running-related injury prevention through innate impact-moderating behaviour', *Medicine and Science in Sports and Exercise* 21, (1989), pp.130–139.

5 Clarke et al, 'Effects of shoe cushioning upon ground reaction forces in running, *International Journal of Sports Medicine* 4, (1983), pp.247–251.

6 Anthony, (1987) 'The functional anatomy of the running training shoe', *Chiropodist*, (December 1987), pp.451–459.

7 Warburton, *Sportscience* 5 (3), (2001).

8 Bergmann, Kniggendorf, et al, 'Influence of shoes and heel strike on the loading of the hip joint', *Journal of Biomechanics* 28, (1995), pp.817–827.

9 Robbins and Hanna, 'Running-related injury prevention through barefoot adaptations', *Medicine and Science in Sports and Exercise* 19 (1987), pp.148–156.

10 Dyson et al *Equine Veterinary Journal*, 37 (2) (2005), pp.113–121.

11 Rooney, *The Lame Horse*, The Russell Meerdink Company Limited (Winsconsin) 1998.

12 Budiansky, *The Nature of Horses*, Orion Publishing (London) 1997, pp.26–28.

13 MacLeod, *The Truth About Feeding Your Horse*, J.A. Allen (London) 2007, pp.31–32.

14 National Research Council, *Nutrient Requirements of Horses* (6th revised edn), National Academy Press (USA) 2007, p.80.

15 National Research Council, *Nutrient Requirements of Horses* (6th revised edn), National Academy Press (USA) 2007, p.296.

16 National Research Council, *Nutrient Requirements of Horses* (6th revised edn), National Academy Press (USA) 2007, p.98.

17 National Research Council, *Nutrient Requirements of Horses* (6th revised edn), National Academy Press (USA) 2007, p.249.

18 National Research Council, *Nutrient Requirements of Horses* (6th revised edn), National Academy Press (USA) 2007, p.80.

19 Dean, *The Magnesium Miracle*, Random House Publishing Group (New York) 2007, p.244.

20 Dean, *The Magnesium Miracle*, Random House Publishing Group (New York) 2007, p.241.

21 National Research Council, *Nutrient Requirements of Horses* (6th revised edn), National Academy Press (USA) 2007, p.79.

22 MacLeod, *The Truth About Feeding Your Horse*, J.A. Allen (London) 2007, p.80.

23 NRC National Research Council, *Nutrient Requirements of Horses* (6th revised edn), National Academy Press (USA) 2007, p.213.

24 Geor, R., Lecture on insulin resistance 2007.

25 Deacon and Williams, *No Foot, No Horse*, Kenilworth Press (Buckingham) 2002.

Resources

Further reading

Beck, W. and Clayton, H., *Equine Locomotion*, Harcourt Publishers Ltd. (London) 2001.

Bromiley, M., *Equine Injury, Therapy and Rehabilitation*, Blackwell Publishing Ltd. (Oxford) 2007.

Budiansky, S., *The Nature of Horses*, Orion Publishing (London) 1997.

Deacon, M. and Williams, G., *No Foot, No Horse*, Kenilworth Press (Buckingham) 2002.

Dean, C., *The Magnesium Miracle*, Random House Publishing Group (New York) 2007.

Goody, P.C., *Horse Anatomy: A Pictorial Approach to Equine Structures*, J.A. Allen (London) 2004.

Jackson, J., *Founder: Prevention and Care*, Star Ridge Publishing (Harrison, Arkansas) 2001.

—— *Paddock Paradise*, Star Ridge Publishing (Harrison, Arkansas) 2006.

—— *The Horse Owners' Guide to Natural Hoof Care*, Star Ridge Publishing (Harrison, Arkansas) 2002.

—— *The Natural Horse*, Star Ridge Publishing (Harrison, Arkansas) 1998.

MacLeod., C., *The Truth About Feeding Your Horse*, J.A. Allen (London) 2007.

National Research Council, *Nutrient Requirements of Horses* (6th revised edn), National Academy Press (USA) 2007.

Ramey, P., *Making Natural Hoof Care Work for You*, Star Ridge Publishing (Arizona) 2003.

Rooney, J., *The Lame Horse*, The Russell Meerdink Company Limited (Winsconsin) 1998.

Simmonds-Lancaster, L., *The Sound Horse*, Equine Accupressure Inc. (USA) 2004.

Useful websites

www.uknhcp.org UK Natural Hoof Care Practitioners' site

www.performancebarefoot.co.uk Sarah Braithwaite's site

www.rockleyfarm.co.uk Nic Barker's site

www.barefoothorses.co.uk UK barefoot resource site, run by Nic

www.charnwood-milling.co.uk Feed site

www.safergrass.org Katy Watts' US laminitis site

www.equinenutritionist.co.uk Clare Macleod's (nutritionist) site

www.thenaturalhoof.co.uk Julie Bailey's site

www.newc.co.uk National equine welfare council site

www.lantra.co.uk Government body which sets national occupational standards for trimmers and farriers

www.hoofrehab.com Peter Ramey's US site

www.hoofcare.com Hoofcare and Lameness magazine site

www.ironfreehoof.com Paige Poss's US site

www.tribeequus.com Cindy Sullivan's US site

Index